KETO PESCATARIAN DIET FOR BEGINNERS

A Practical Approach for Healthy Diet and Weight Loss with some Amazing Fish and Veggie Recipes

MAYA BRYCE

Table of Contents

1.   INTRODUCTION

You might be surprised to learn that the Ketogenic Pescatarian Diet has been around a long time—about 100 years. It was initially developed to help children who were experiencing seizures.

But what exactly is keto? The basic premise of the Ketogenic Pescatarian Diet is to eat low carb and high fat. This is counterintuitive to many of us who have traditionally been taught that fat is bad for us, and we should certainly not eat much of it if we hope to lose weight. The truth is, though, that by eating enough of the correct types of fat, your body will enter a metabolic state known as "nutritional ketosis." It might seem more than a little crazy to think you can lose fat by eating fat, but the scientific basis is sound. Our bodies mainly run on glucose, which is the product of the breakdown of carbohydrates such as rice, grains, pasta, cereals, etc. But when we drastically reduce our carbohydrate intake and add a high amount of fat to our diet, our bodies switch from using carbohydrates as fuel to using fat as fuel, and we are then able to reach ketosis.

Nutritional ketosis allows your body to become a fat-burning machine by turning fat into ketones in the liver. Ketones are a secondary form of energy that our bodies need to function. This backup fuel system allows us to track our metabolism into burning stored fat rather than carbohydrates. These ketones become the primary source of energy for our organs, muscles, and brain to function correctly. Many researchers believe that ketones are a more efficient fuel source than carbohydrates because they burn more slowly, giving your body a more sustainable source of energy.

The Ketogenic Pescatarian Diet is immensely popular thanks to its wide array of benefits. Various studies show that diet can reduce inflammation, increase energy, decrease food cravings (especially for sugar), help clear skin, improve fat burning, slow the effects of aging, and lower the risk of chronic disease. However, one of the most talked-about advantages to living a keto lifestyle is mental clarity.

Neurological inflammation has been linked to reduced cognitive function, as well as depression and anxiety. Just about everyone who has followed the Ketogenic Pescatarian Diet claims to have experienced the benefit of clearer thinking. An overall inflammation most likely causes neurological inflammation that, in turn, affects the brain by increasing focal brain inflammation.

As mentioned, keto was initially used to treat children with epilepsy. Since then, it has proved effective in battling severe illnesses such as diabetes, Parkinson's, and autoimmune diseases, including Hashimoto's. The diet has been shown to increase glutathione, a combination of amino acids that's your body's most potent detoxifier (and something often found lacking in people with autoimmune issues). While in nutritional ketosis, your body will naturally produce more glutathione, which acts as a powerful antioxidant that reduces oxidative stress caused by a poor diet, anxiety, or infection.

Weight loss is also a result of eating a ketogenic diet, and it often happens quickly. Fundamentally, when you starve your body of carbs and sugar, your blood sugar decreases. Your body responds by switching to the alternate form of energy—ketones—and then for as long as you stay in ketosis, your body will continue to burn fat. It is not uncommon for people to lose most of their unwanted pounds in the early stages of keto, while others experience a steady weight loss for as long as they are in ketosis.

Macros, which is short for macronutrients, refers to the three primary nutrients our bodies need to function: protein, fats, and carbohydrates. Your body converts these nutrients into energy for your brain, muscles, and organs. In most diets, macros are tailored toward a person's body type, activity level, and nutritional needs. For example, some foods recommend a 30 percent fat, 35 percent protein, and 35 percent carbohydrate split of daily calories. Pescatarian ketogenic macros, on the other hand, typically target 70 percent fat, 20 percent protein, and 10 percent net carbs, most of those carbs coming from vegetables.

You may have seen the terms "total carbs" and "net carbs" on food labels. "Total carbs" is the tally of all the sugars, fiber, and indigestible starch in a food item. Our bodies need a tissue to be able to excrete waste products efficiently, but because we cannot digest fiber, it does not affect blood sugar levels. "Net carbs" refer to the carbohydrates that can be converted into sugar in our bodies and therefore affect blood sugar levels.

When calculating net carbs, it's essential to ignore sugar alcohols. These are organic compounds found in vegetables, fruit, and many sugar-free products. They have a much lower impact on blood sugar than regular sugars, which is why they are typically subtracted when calculating net carbs. Here's the formula:

Total carbohydrates − fiber − sugar alcohols = net carbs

While you are on the ketogenic diet, you will want to pay attention to the foods you buy to make sure you keep within the 10 percent carbohydrate ratio for your total overall daily calories. The good news is that you don't need to carry around a calculator to track your macros on the keto diet. There are several helpful apps (available for a small monthly fee) that you can customize for individual macro percentages. Some of my favorites are MyFitnessPal, Calorie King, and Carb Manager. You may also find it helpful to keep a food journal, at least until you become accustomed to the diet.

As mentioned, many people associate the keto diet with having to consume a great deal of meat, particularly fatty steak and bacon. Not enough studies have been done to calculate the health risks of such high meat consumption on a long-term basis. Even if you're not a Pescatarian, you may have come to this book because you're curious about the Ketogenic Pescatarian Diet and eager to try it for its multiple benefits, but you are concerned about the diet's overreliance on meat consumption. The good news is that a Pescatarian keto diet is possible and comes with its own set of benefits.

Most Pescatarian s rely heavily on carbohydrates such as beans, rice, pasta, and bread to keep them full. One challenge of following the ketogenic Pescatarian diet, therefore, is figuring out how to replace those carbs with a higher amount of fat and protein. Fortunately, if you're already a plant-based eater, you're likely used to alternative forms of protein such as edamame, tofu, eggs, and some dairy products. Switching from using carbs for fuel to using fat should be reasonably easy for you since you are already comfortable with making substitutions.

People decide to adopt a Ketogenic Pescatarian Diet for different reasons, whether it is to manage their blood sugar better, to lose weight, or even to reduce dependence on certain prescription medications. All of these benefits can come from eating keto. Plant-based diets have some pretty incredible benefits as well, including lowering high blood pressure, keeping cholesterol in check, and reducing overall inflammation that can be caused by animal proteins. So, it only makes sense to combine the Pescatarian and ketogenic diets into one super diet.

2. THE BASICS OF THE KETO DIET

This will highlight the necessary information needed before starting the ketogenic diet. Understanding the main principles of keto, how it works, and steps to take before starting will ensure a more successful experience! The keto diet offers numerous benefits that will also be outlined in this.

1. What Is Keto?

The ketogenic weight loss plan, or keto for short, is a diet that makes a specialty of ingesting little to no carbs, however excessive quantities of fat.

The result of eating in such a manner forces the frame right into a metabolic state called ketosis. During ketosis, the structure makes use of fat as energy due to the absence of carbs. Typically, glucose is the primary supply of energy. Glucose is derived from carbs.

The fats consumed through food are used as energy, but ketosis is also successful in using fat stores in the body as well. This process is compelling for those looking to lose high amounts of body fat. The process starts in the liver, where the body converts fat into ketones. Ketones are what replace or act like glucose while you follow the keto diet. Ketones are always present when in ketosis. In simple terms, when the body is in ketosis, ketones are being used as energy instead of glucose.

Although there are many different keto diet versions, the standard keto diet or SKD is the most popular. Other versions are supervised by health professionals or used by athletes. All versions of the keto diet rely on the same concepts but may alter carbohydrate levels based on unique circumstances. An SKD diet is classified as 75% fat, 20% protein, and only 5% carbs (Freeman, Kossoff, & Hartman, 2007). Because the Keto diet has strict macronutrient intake, many foods are eliminated. However, much of the keto diet's success comes from consuming an average number of calories. So, the keto diet does not restrict calories but does mostly limit the type of foods that can be eaten. Many diets fail because the temptations of overeating are too high. With the keto diet, you'll never go hungry, and many modifications can be made so the same foods can be enjoyed.

2. What Are the Benefits of Keto?

One of the main reasons many start the keto diet is to lose weight. The Ketogenic Pescatarian Diet has become well known and popular among many due to its ability to shed a large number of pounds, fast. A study found that those on the keto diet lost 2.2 times more weight than those on a calorie-restricted, low-fat diet (Brehm et al., 2003). As mentioned, part of the success of the keto diet is its no restrictiveness in terms of calories. Feeling full and satisfied is allowed and also encouraged. Eating lots of healthy fats provides a sense of comfort, but it also helps keep energy levels up. On calorie-restricting diets, lethargic and binge-eats are common because the body always feels like it's missing something. The keto diet allows fat loss without restricting or controlling food, making the menu more suitable for everyday life. Food elimination is essential, while restricting calories is not.

Other reasons the keto diet is successful for weight loss has to do with hormones. Leptin and ghrelin, known as the hunger hormones, see a positive change while on the keto diet. Leptin is a hormone made by fat cells that decreases appetite, while ghrelin is the opposite (ghrelin will increase appetite). Both play a crucial role in weight management. Both hormones must maintain a healthy balance, so the brain knows when to stop eating, and your body feels satisfied sooner. Diets that are high in sugar and carbs may trigger leptin resistance, which hinders the brain from feeling full. Leptin resistance is a problem because the brain doesn't know when to stop eating or see when the body is starving. Cloudy signals lead to overeating and a false sense of hunger. According to Perfect Keto (2019), the keto diet decreases ghrelin levels, reduces hunger, and regulates leptin. A controlled appetite, increased satiety and fat burning, higher leptin sensitivity, and the prevention of insulin resistance are the scientific reasons the keto diet is excellent for weight loss.

The keto food plan is frequently advocated for those suffering from type diabetes and for prediabetics. Diabetes is diagnosed as adjustments within the metabolism, high blood sugar, and impaired insulin function. Insulin is a hormone made within the pancreas regulating blood sugar stages from getting too excessive or low. Insulin can be the central aspect of weight gain or excess fat storage. When the frame doesn't respond to insulin, extra is produced. This can be brought about by sugar, carbs, an unhealthy lifestyle, or lack of exercise. However, I have a look at located that the keto weight-reduction plan progressed insulin sensitivity by way of 75% (Boden et al., 2005)! The examination suggests that many had been capable of forestalling the usage of all diabetes medications. (However, before you anticipate your prescription, get permitted from your physician first!) The weight loss plan's capacity to enhance insulin sensitivity has proven helpful for type two diabetes and prediabetic situations.

Other conditions have additionally shown advantageous modifications when uncovered to a ketogenic lifestyle. Those situations include but aren't restricted to coronary heart disease, positive cancers, Alzheimer's disease, epilepsy, Parkinson's disease, polycystic ovary syndrome, mind injuries, and acne (Mawer, 2020).

In everyday life, the keto diet offers increased energy and focus. Many report feelings of mental clarity, improved concentration, and higher energy levels while on the keto diet. Fortunately, there is no placebo effect when it comes to these feelings because all three are backed by science. The simple explanation is that ketones are a better source of energy than glucose, as ketones can carry more energy per unit when combined with oxygen than glucose (Fan, 2013). This means that when oxygen is breathed in, a more significant response occurs when the oxygen reaches a ketone than glucose. This stimulates and creates a more substantial response from the brain and translates into various mental benefits. From a cellular perspective, the mitochondria in brain cells receive more oxygen when ketones are present, which produces more brain activity.

In summary, the keto diet offers many health benefits and has shown improvements in certain diseases or medical conditions. Whether starting the diet to lose weight or manage a condition, rest assured there are benefits for all.

Starting a new diet or lifestyle can be challenging. However, the keto diet is one of the easiest to implement. With that being said, there are a few steps to take beforehand to maximize success.

The first step is to prepare for the changes coming mentally. It's essential to make and visualize the journey ahead psychologically. For many, writing down goals and aspirations proves helpful. Avoiding foods or unhealthy habits you once enjoyed will be even more complicated if the end goals are not clear. During this step, write down all of the reasons a change is necessary. After reading about the benefits, be sure to include which apply most and are the most intriguing. If the main goal is to lose weight, write down all the desired outcomes, and how you will feel once that goal is achieved.

Once a list has been prepared, put it in a safe place to reference when times get hard. It's also recommended to keep a weekly blog. It will be easier to make adjustments for quicker results, but your progress can be tracked. Seeing the positive changes from week to week is encouraging! Not all changes will be physical, so a short entry detailing other positive changes is necessary. Staying in tune with goals weekly and monitoring the positive changes will help you to keep going!

Related to the above, before you start keto, it is also recommended to go for a check-up with your health care provider and run some simple blood work for cholesterol, creatinine, a complete blood count, your fasting blood glucose, and hemoglobin A1c (Bourdua-Roy et al., n.d.). These results are essential as low-carb diets can have adverse indications, and these can only be seen when you visit the lab and get the results. Ideally, get your types of blood tested every three months.

The second step is to consider telling a close friend or partner all the goals you wish to achieve. An accountability partner may be helpful but isn't necessary if you feel uncomfortable. Talking with an accountability partner or someone in a similar situation can increase motivation. Sharing frustrations or goals is healthy for mental health and creates a release that subdues stress.

Lifestyle changes aren't always easy, and sharing wins and defeats can make the journey easier. If you're comfortable sharing your lifestyle change, it may be easier to stick to the keto guidelines and avoid temptations in social settings. However, not all situations will prompt questions from others, and most of the time, many won't notice the skipped treat or breadstick. Step one will be of extra benefit if you prefer to keep your changes private.

The third step to take before starting the keto diet is cleaning out the pantry or rearranging. If you're living with others, it might not be possible to get rid of treats or temptations. Consider keeping your food in a unique location where other people's diet isn't visible. For example, your pantry can be created and does not have to be in a traditional "pantry" location. In the refrigerator, keep your food organized and in one place. This will help prevent the urge to cheat or binge. The keto diet is safe and healthy for most, and the entire household/family can participate. For example, chips, bread, treats, and more can still be enjoyed with some modifications. Replace unhealthy foods with keto-approved foods. If you're living alone or making the lifestyle change with your partner, donate the unhealthy foods and get them out of sight! If you're able, control what foods are in the house, so fewer temptations are possible.

By taking these three steps, your chances of a successful keto diet will increase. Staying focused and persistent will yield results! Don't forget to track your progress and make adjustments as necessary.

3. WHY CHOOSE THE KETO LIFESTYLE?

There are many blessings to the ketogenic weight loss plan, including increased energy, weight loss, and both the remedy and prevention of many diseases. In this, we will discuss a number of the most commonplace motives to select the ketogenic eating regimen and the health-promoting qualities it could provide.

3. Weight Loss

While science has shown that BMI has little merit and you can be both fat and healthy, and there is no shame in being fat and proud even if you are unhealthy, there is still much scientific backing showing that having a higher body fat percentage increases your risk of disease. Many people may try crash diets to lower their weight, but years of these diets take a toll on your health and reduce your metabolism and make it more challenging to lose weight over time. You often even gain the weight back soon after quitting the diet.

Thankfully, the Ketogenic Pescatarian Diet is not a fad diet; it's been proven to be healthy, and it supports maintainable weight loss. Rather than starving your body of calories and nutrients, you can provide it with ample energy, vitamins, and minerals while enjoying a variety of natural and delicious meals.

When you are on a standard high-carbohydrate diet, the constant assault of carbohydrates on your body causes an insulin and blood sugar response. It prevents your body from burning off the digested fat and body fat. Yet when you are on a low-carbohydrate and high-fat diet, your body is burning off fat by default. Not only will it burn off the fat you consume, but it will also burn off your body fat and increase your metabolism, helping you to lose weight.

The rate of your weight loss can be customized, depending on how much of a caloric deficit you are eating. It is unhealthy to lose more than two to three pounds a week, so if after the first two weeks of the Ketogenic Pescatarian Diet, you are losing more than this, then adjust your caloric deficit so that you are losing weight at a slightly slower pace. Though you may lose quite a bit the first couple of weeks in water weight, this should not concern you.

Need to gain weight, you can accomplish that on the Ketogenic Pescatarian Diet by merely adjusting your caloric intake. Some people may consume twelve-hundred calories a day; others may consume sixteen-hundred, while others are two-thousand. It all depends on the needs of your body, your doctor's recommendations, and whether or not you have an eating disorder.

4. Lower Your Cholesterol

We are used to hearing about how bad fats are for us, causing disease, and clog our arteries. Since the war on fat in the 1990s and early 2000s, people have been afraid of fat, even from health sources. While there was a little truth to this, certain fats, such as trans fats, are bad for you, and there are many healthy fats. Yet fats such as those found in avocados, olives, sesame seeds, coconut, and nuts have been found to have fantastic health benefits and weight loss promoting qualities. The Ketogenic Pescatarian Diet and these healthy sources of fats have been shown to lower dangerous cholesterol, increase healthy cholesterol, and reduce the risk of developing cardiovascular diseases.

If you have heard about the Ketogenic Pescatarian Diet raising cholesterol, it was most likely a misunderstanding, as this has never been shown to be true. On the contrary, multiple studies have shown the cholesterol-lowering properties of the ketogenic diet. The good cholesterol, which the Ketogenic Pescatarian Diet does raise, is necessary to lower bad cholesterol. This type of cholesterol boosts vitamin D absorption, manages hormones, and aids in the digestion of food. Good cholesterol, known as HDL, is entirely harmless and promotes increased health.

There are two types of dangerous cholesterol, not one. These are LDL and the lesser-known VLDL. These cause a buildup of plaque in the arteries and increase the risk of a heart attack. On one study of the ketogenic diet, sixty-six obese patients who experienced high cholesterol went on the Ketogenic Pescatarian Diet and were able to lose weight, increase good cholesterol, lower bad cholesterol, as well as blood glucose and triglycerides. The study was deemed successful and that the Ketogenic Pescatarian Diet was shown to be a valuable treatment against high cholesterol and heart disease.

5. Reduce Aging

The mitochondrial cells can utilize amino acids, fatty acids, and glucose for fuel. These cells are required to produce ninety percent of the energy our body needs, and we are unable to survive without them. If these cells are not thriving, then neither can we.

While incredibly powerful and necessary, sometimes while converting fuel into energy for our cells, electrons can escape. This process will cause dangerous free radicals to form, and worse yet, these are the most dangerous type of free radicals, known as reactive oxygen species.

While this process is a natural part of aging and happens without most people being aware, it does cause cellular damage and degradation. Thankfully, the Ketogenic Pescatarian Diet can fight against this process by increasing the number of mitochondrial cells, increasing the cell's ability to convert energy efficiently. It contains many powerful antioxidants that neutralize and remove these free radicals. This not only slows down the aging of your skin but your entire body and mind.

The Ketogenic Pescatarian Diet has impressive benefits for treating seizures, both those caused by epilepsy and those that are not. The Ketogenic Pescatarian Diet was created nearly one-hundred years ago to treat epilepsy before anticonvulsants were created. While the Ketogenic Pescatarian Diet declined with the discovery of anticonvulsant drugs, it made a resurgence once people realized that drugs are ineffective in many people. While the Ketogenic Pescatarian Diet alone is not for everyone with uncontrolled epilepsy, it has been shown to reduce seizures in many cases significantly. This is especially great as anticonvulsants have a high rate of side effects, including drowsiness, sleepiness, and mental fatigue. These symptoms get in the way of life and even many people's jobs, making it hard to stay on the anticonvulsants, also if needed. Thankfully, the Ketogenic Pescatarian Diet provides people with more options.

There have been countless studies demonstrating the success of treating seizures and epilepsy with the ketogenic diet. In one study that took place at Trinity College between 2001 and 2006, there were one-hundred and forty-five participants. All of these participants were resistant to drug therapy in the past. Out of these patients, seven percent experienced a reduction of more than ninety percent in seizure activity. Thirty-eight percent of the people experienced an improvement of over fifty percent reduction in seizure activity.

While for most people on the ketogenic diet, the body will provide enough ketones for their needs, those with neurological and neurodegenerative diseases may want to boost their ketones, even more, to protect their brains from potential damage caused by the illness. In this case, MCT oil (medium-chain triglycerides) and exogenous ketones have been found to provide benefits and further reduce seizure activity. While some children who have sensitive stomachs may not be able to handle the ketogenic diet, while not as effective, MCT and exogenous ketones along may provide a small amount of benefit. This is because both of these products increase the number of ketones available to protect the brain; therefore, preventing seizures.

While most of our cells can use ketones as a fuel source rather than glucose, this is not true of cancer and tumor cells. This means that when you are on the ketogenic diet, the meager amount of glucose in your body and the production of ketones can starve cancer and tumor cells of energy to grow. Some studies have shown that within a few days of beginning the ketogenic diet, tumor cells, whether cancerous or not, have been shown to start shrinking. It has also been shown to halt tumor growth, improve symptoms, and increase the effectiveness of chemotherapy. All of these benefits from the Ketogenic Pescatarian Diet for treating cancer are reversed if the person discontinues the ketogenic diet.

Age-related diseases have dramatically increased over the years, and Alzheimer's is the most common and debilitating of these diseases. Startling, there are nearly forty-four million people worldwide who have either Alzheimer's disease or related dementia, and out of these people,

Alzheimer's Disease International estimates that one in four will be diagnosed.

Not only is this disease severe on the person diagnosed, but on the family as well. It takes a toll on the family's emotions, time, and finances, but in 2016, 15.9 million family members provided care at an estimated 18.2 billable hours, which is 240 billion dollars.

The worst news is that Alzheimer's disease is the sixth leading cause of death in the United States, and typical life expectancy after diagnosis is only four to eight years. Startlingly, between the years of 2000 and 2014, there was an eighty-nine percent increase in deaths from Alzheimer's disease, and it is estimated that between 2017 and 2025, there will be a 14% increase in the condition.

This disease causes the neurons in the brain to develop insulin resistance, making it difficult for them to absorb glucose and therefore stave for fuel. Thankfully, not only do ketones act as a non-glucose fuel source for these cells, but the diet has also been shown to decrease insulin resistance. This will provide the cells with ketones for fuel, but by treating the insulin resistance, they will better be able to absorb the glucose that is offered to them through the gluconeogenesis process.

One study was conducted on twenty adult participants who lived with either Alzheimer's or other cognitive impairment diseases. In this study, the participants were given either an MCT oil drink, which increases ketone levels or a placebo. Within ninety minutes of drinking the MCT drink, people's ketones increased significantly, and they displayed significant improvements in symptoms, whereas the placebo-control group did not improve.

In another study, a patient with Alzheimer's disease went on a treatment protocol with coconut oil and MCT oil for twenty months. The patient experienced significant improvement and success. They improved fourteen points on the scale of Activities of Daily Living and six points on the Alzheimer's Disease Assessment Scale-Cognitive. The patient experienced a remarkable improvement in mood, word-finding, recalling events, social participation, tremors, and gait during this time. MRI scans conducted throughout the test period displayed that his brain experienced no decline during the twenty-month treatment period.

A study that compared the effects of high-carbohydrate diets and low-carbohydrate diets on senior adults found that the participants on a low-carbohydrate diet showed improved functioning. These patients experienced a loss in fat around the abdomen and weight loss, as well as enhanced fasting insulin, memory performance, and fasting glucose. This improvement was concluded to be the result of increased ketones from the diet.

4. WHO IS A PESCATARIAN?

A pescatarian is someone that includes fish to their diet but avoids meat and other poultry. The term was coined in the early 1990s with a combination of two words, 'Pesce,' which means fish, and 'vegetarian.' In summary, a pescatarian is anyone who follows the vegetarian diet, but also includes fish and other seafood to his or her diet. The menu is mainly made up of plant-based foods like legumes, healthy fats, nuts, whole grains, and produce, with seafood being the primary protein source.

It may interest you to know that several pescatarians eat eggs and dairy too. In the same way that we have several versions of the vegetarian diet, we also have several versions of the pescatarian diet. One can eat a diet free of meat but packed with plenty of junk foods, processed starches, and fish sticks instead of a healthier diet.

6. What do Pescatarians Eat?

- Peanuts and seeds, nuts and nut butter
- Whole grains and grain products
- Vegetables
- Fruits
- Seeds including flaxseeds, chia, and hemp
- Legumes including lentils, hummus, tofu and beans
- Dairy including cheese, milk, and yogurt
- Shellfish and fish
- Eggs
- What not to Eat
- Pork
- Turkey
- Chicken
- Beef

- Lamb
- Wild game
-

7. What Did a Pescatarian Eat?

Pesce means "fish" in Italian, so it's easy to conclude that a pescatarian is a vegetarian who eats fish. But is it that simple? Well, sort of. To make sure we're clear and not missing any of the incredible food groups available in the pescatarian lifestyle, here's an overview of the foods pescatarians eat.

Beans, lentils, and legumes. This category also includes soy products like edamame, tofu, and tempeh. And don't forget chickpeas, which make delectable hummus.

Eggs. Pescatarians differ on eggs—some choose to eat them, some omit them. It's up to you.

Dairy products. As with eggs, some pescatarians eat milk, cheese, yogurt, kefir, and other dairy products, whereas others avoid these foods.

Fruits.

Nuts and seeds. These can be used in a medley of ways to add an abundance of exciting and intriguing flavors and textures to your meals and snacks.

Seafood. Any fish or shellfish that comes from a river, lake, bay, or ocean is fair for a pescatarian.

Vegetables. There's no chance of boredom with the full range of colors, textures, and flavors available from plants!

Whole grains. When paired with other plant-based foods, whole grains like barley, rice, oats, and bread can help create complete proteins, which are essential for people following a mostly plant-based diet.

8. What Doesn't a Pescatarian Eat?

Though it may go without saying, here's a look at what you'll be leaving off the grocery list when you convert to a pescatarian lifestyle:

Organ meat. Avoid all organ meats and offal—including liver, tongue, sweetbreads, tripe, and chitterlings.

Red meat. Pescatarians avoid all meats that come from mammals and are red in their raw state (beef, lamb, pork, veal, venison, etc.).

Wild game. Although less popular than red meat and white meat, game meats—including pheasant, rabbit, venison, and wild boar—won't make an appearance on a pescatarian's plate.

White meat. Poultry, such as chicken, duck, goose, and turkey, are also off-limits.

9. Reasons to Change Your Lifestyle

Perhaps you've been an omnivore and are now eliminating meat and poultry from your diet. Or maybe you were a vegetarian and are now reintroducing fish. Here are just a few reasons for choosing a pescatarian lifestyle.

Additional health benefits. Eating less red meat has been shown to lower the risks of developing high blood pressure, heart disease, and cancer. As a pescatarian, you'll consume less saturated fat and experience the benefits of healthy fats found in plant-based food sources and heart-healthy omega-3 fatty acids found in fish, such as salmon and mackerel.

Environmental concerns. Omitting meat from your diet may also be a way to reduce your carbon footprint due to the abundance of natural resources it takes to raise land animals.

Variety. If you've been a vegetarian, adding fish to your diet means more variety in flavor and more sources of essential nutrients, like iron, vitamin B12, and protein.

Weight loss. Omitting red meat, poultry, wild game, and organ meat from your diet means you'll likely be eating a higher amount of nutrient-dense and low-calorie plant-based foods than before, which are generally also lower in calories. Plus, enjoying a variety of seafood will help keep the process from feeling too restrictive.

10. Reasons to Follow a Pescatarian Diet

Several people follow the pescatarian diet for different reasons. Some of these reasons are:

Health benefits

Research has proven that plant-based diets have several advantages, including lowering the risk of obesity and chronic diseases like diabetes and heart disease. Research also shows that you can get these protective benefits from following the pescatarian diet.

One study proved that women who followed the pescatarian diet gained 2.5 fewer pounds than women who had meat in their food. Also, people who changed their diet to plant-based gained the least amount of weight. This means that reducing your consumption of meat and poultry may be beneficial to your health regardless of your current eating patterns.

Another study concluded that people on a pescatarian diet had reduced the risk of developing diabetes at 4.8 percent compared to omnivores at 7.6 percent.

Also, one study looked at people who were pescatarian or rarely ate meat. It discovered that these people had a 22 percent lower risk of dying from heart diseases than people who eat meat regularly.

Environmental concerns

United Nations quoted that raising livestock contributes to 15 percent of all human-made carbon emissions. While producing fish and other seafood generates lower carbon than any animal meat or cheese.

One study conducted in 2014 calculated that fish eaters' diets caused 46 percent less greenhouse gas emissions than that of people who consumed at least one serving of meat each day.

Ethical reasons

Some people may choose to be vegetarians for ethical reasons, and the same applies to pescatarians. Some ethical reasons for which people may prefer to avoid meat in their diet include:

Inhumane factory practices: they are not in support of factory farms that raise livestock in harsh and inhumane conditions.

Opposing slaughter: they do not support the killing of animals for food.

Humanitarian reasons: they believe producing grain to feed to animals is a waste of resources and land, considering the world's level of hunger.

Poor labor conditions: they do not want to be a part of factory farms that poorly treat their workers.

11. The Health Benefits of a Pescatarian Lifestyle

The way you feed your body can have a significant impact on your overall health. If you stick to a pescatarian eating plan, you will get all the benefits of a plant-based diet with the additional protein and nutrients of seafood. Plus, you'll eliminate the risks associated with eating meat. Here's just a taste of the benefits you could experience.

Brain health. We all want healthy brains. Studies suggest eating fish may support this. A 2016 study showed that eating at least three servings of fish per week while you're pregnant could benefit your offspring's brain. Research also shows that eating fish can lower the risk of developing Alzheimer's disease.

Heart health. Opting for a pescatarian diet can be a way to nourish your heart. Oily fish, such as mackerel and salmon, are rich in omega-3 fatty acids, which have been shown to reduce the risk of fatal heart attacks and congestive heart failure. And studies have shown that people who follow a plant-based diet are less likely to develop coronary heart disease.

Inflammation. Inflammation is associated with some diseases, and many of the foods in a pescatarian diet star in an anti-inflammatory diet, especially fatty fish, which are rich in omega-3 fats.

Minimizing cancer risk, limiting your intake of red meats and processed meats can reduce your risk of developing certain cancers.

Weight loss. As mentioned earlier, those who follow a pescatarian diet can maintain or lose weight because of the lower calories and higher nutrient density of the foods most frequently eaten in this lifestyle.

12. Benefits of Adding Fish to a Diet

You will enjoy several benefits when you add fish to the vegetarian diet. Several people are worried that avoiding animal flesh or eliminating animal products could cause a low intake of certain vital nutrients. For instance, it is tough to get protein, calcium, zinc, and vitamin B12 on a vegan diet. When you add seafood like mollusks, crustaceans, and fish to the vegetarian diet, you will begin to enjoy your diet's vital nutrients and varieties.

Get more omega-3s

The better manner to get omega-three fatty acids is by ingesting fish. Some plant-based foods like flaxseed walnuts contain alpha-linolenic acid, which is a type of omega-3 fat. But it is not easy for the body to convert this type of acid to docosahexaenoic acid DHA and eicosapentaenoic acid (EPA). EPA and DHA have more benefits that are helpful to the heart, brain, and mood. Oily fish like sardines and salmon contain both DHA and EPA.

Boost your protein intake

Every person needs a daily intake of about 0.8g of protein per 2.2 pounds of body weight to stay healthy. So, a person who weighs 150 pounds needs to eat a minimum of 54 grams of protein daily. It can be tough to achieve a high protein diet with just plant-based foods, particularly if you do not want extra fat or carbs with your protein. An excellent source of lean protein is fish and other seafood, as it gives your body the protein needed for the body to perform optimally.

Seafood has other nutrients

Apart from protein and omega-3s, seafood is rich in several other nutrients. For example, oysters have a high content of vitamin B12, selenium, and zinc. One oyster gives 55 percent of the RDI for selenium and zinc, as well as 133 percent of the RDI for vitamin B12.

Mussel is another seafood with high contents of selenium, manganese, vitamin B12, and other B vitamins.

Whitefish varieties like flounder and cod do not have many omega-3 fats but provide extremely lean protein. For instance, 3 ounces of cod produces less than a gram of fat and 19 grams of protein. Cod is an excellent choice for people who need niacin, phosphorus, selenium, vitamins B6 and vitamins B12

Gives you more options

The vegetarian diet can be limiting at times, especially when eating out at restaurants. If you eat food to stay healthy, then being a pescatarian offers you more meal options. And fish makes a good option as you can prepare it in several ways; grill, bake or sauté.

5.   THE PESCATARIAN DIET

To get commenced on our pescatarian weight loss program journey, we want to learn more about it. Pesce is Italian for "fish." A pescatarian food plan is much like a Mediterranean weight loss program, or to a vegetarian food regimen with the addition of fish and seafood. This eating fashion emphasizes minimally processed components and whole-food resources for carbohydrates, protein, and fat. Here are some of the other defining capabilities of this style of eating:

Living in Seattle—home of the famous Pike Place Market fish throwers and many Alaskan fisherpersons and seafood processors—I've always been lucky to have access to incredible seafood. Perhaps that, along with growing up in a Norwegian American family, has contributed to my love of seafood. I hope to share that enthusiasm with you in the that follow. Being a pescatarian may feel restrictive because you are no longer eating red meat or poultry, but I promise you won't feel deprived. Changing your lifestyle also comes with a learning curve. I am excited to share with you the tips and tricks I've gathered from personal experience to help you in your journey to becoming—and staying—a pescatarian.

The 5 Major Principles of The Pescatarian Diet

If you're new to a pescatarian lifestyle, there are several vital components to remember. Although there are many variety and flexibility in this style of eating, some of the most common features are listed below.

Fish and Seafood as Primary Animal Proteins: A pescatarian diet includes fresh and saltwater fish, shellfish, and crustaceans. You won't see ingredients such as beef, pork, poultry, wild game, or other meats.

The Ability to Include Eggs and Dairy: Many pescatarians choose to include eggs and dairy as protein sources. However, some prefer to rely solely on fish and seafood for animal protein. The best part about the pescatarian diet is that the choice is up to you.

Plant-Forward Focus: Many people gravitate toward plant-based eating for health or environmental concerns. A pescatarian diet is similar in that regard and can offer a realistic compromise for people who don't want to go entirely vegetarian.

Lots of Fruits and Vegetables: A pescatarian diet encourages a high intake of fruits and vegetables. These are nutrient-rich ingredients that provide many essential vitamins and minerals and beneficial antioxidants and phytochemicals for health.

Whole Grains and Fiber-Rich Foods: A pescatarian diet is not meant to be a low-carbohydrate diet. It includes carbohydrates from whole grains and other starchy or fiber-rich foods such as potatoes, legumes, and ancient grains.

10 Common Questions About a Pescatarian Diet

It's not unusual to have questions or concerns about adding more fish to your diet. I hope you could read below to learn some of the most common questions I hear as a dietitian.

Will a pescatarian diet help me lose weight?

While there are many ways a pescatarian diet can help you improve health, it is not a weight-loss diet. Weight is not a controllable behavior. We can, however, support good health by eating balanced, nourishing meals. Adopting a pescatarian diet as part of your lifestyle may lead to improvements in health, including some potential weight loss, but weight loss is not guaranteed or our primary goal.

Can I substitute other proteins instead of seafood?

Although a right pescatarian diet doesn't include beef, poultry, pork, or other meats, many families enjoy these foods regardless. This book was written to help you adopt the diet, but if you want to swap out seafood for other animal proteins every once in a while, that is okay. It would be best if you did not eat seafood every day

Should I eat seafood every day?

No. The current recommendation for adults is two to three servings per week (totaling eight to 12 ounces). A pescatarian diet does not require you to include seafood at every meal; in fact, most of your meals could be plant-based.

Is a pescatarian diet safe?

A pescatarian diet is safe for most people, so long as you're aware of which fish contain high levels of mercury. Generally, the higher the fish appears on the food chain, the higher the mercury content. Some of the highest-mercury fish include swordfish, shark, king mackerel, and tilefish. Additionally, pregnant women should avoid more than six ounces of albacore (white) tuna. Pregnant women should also avoid raw fish to reduce the risk of foodborne illness.

Do I have to include eggs or dairy?

Many people who identify as pescatarians include eggs and dairy, but it is a personal choice. There are limitations for someone with lactose intolerance or an allergy to eggs or dairy. In those cases, many alternative products can be used in recipes as a replacement, such as a nut or coconut kinds of milk.

Can I get enough protein on a pescatarian diet?

Yes. Most adults in the United States are easily able to meet the recommended amounts of protein each day. Because a pescatarian diet includes protein from fish and seafood, plant-based protein from various sources, and the option to add eggs and dairy products, there are few concerns about protein intake for those following the diet.

Will I be able to afford the ingredients needed to make these recipes or follow the meal plan?

These recipes include affordable options that are easy to find in most grocery stores. Some types of seafood can be quite expensive, but these recipes are built around fresh or frozen fillets of commonly available fish or canned options for tuna and salmon. There are also tips included for ingredient substitutions if you are unable to find or purchase ingredients called for in a recipe. And because a pescatarian diet doesn't require seafood in every meal, you can further stretch your grocery budget by relying on plant-based meals when you choose to skip seafood.

How long will I have to spend cooking?

Many of the recipes can be made in 30 minutes or less and are labeled as such. If you have even less time, look for the Quick Prep label for meals that require little or no active cooking and take 10 minutes or less to prepare. Some meals, such as slow cooker meals and recipes that need time to chill or freeze, may take longer overall, but the active preparation time will not belong.

 How can I make a pescatarian diet more family-friendly?

Introducing any new foods to family meals can be challenging. However, these recipes feature familiar flavors and can be easily modified to fit your family's tastes. Seafood is safe to introduce to infants 6 to 12 months of age, but if you have concerns about food allergies or your child is prone to them, please consult with your pediatrician and dietitian first. As for serving family-friendly pescatarian meals, you can plate ingredients separately, use spices and seasonings more sparingly, or offer dipping sauces or other condiments to appeal to younger children's tastes. For more information on family meals, I recommend resources by Ellyn Satter, including her Division of Responsibilities model of family feeding.

Will a pescatarian diet harm the environment?

If you are conscious about selecting a variety of sustainably caught or farmed seafood, the inclusion of seafood to your diet should not negatively impact the environment. See the on Eco-friendly Fish for more information to guide your decisions.

6. PREPARING YOUR PESCATARIAN KITCHEN

As a dietitian, one of my favorite catchphrases is "Proper planning provides for peak performance!" While it may be hard to say that five times fast, it couldn't be more accurate than when developing healthy eating habits, like adopting the pescatarian diet.

Without preparation, it's easy to make excuses. Think about it—how many times have you said something like "I don't have beans [or insert any pantry item], so I can't make the bean tacos [or any recipe] I planned. I'll just order takeout instead." One missed dinner turns into two, which turns into several. You forget to restock your pantry, and over time you begin to feel the effects of too much takeout. You're lethargic, bloated from excess salt, and even pack on a few unwanted pounds.

Instead, be prepared for success on the pescatarian diet: stock your pantry, take inventory, and get organized. This way, you'll feel confident in what you're doing. Having a well-stocked kitchen and pantry helps eliminate common obstacles and improves your organization. Frequently used ingredients will be available, you'll cut trips to the supermarket in half, and you'll save time and money. Even more, studies show that being organized can help improve your healthy eating habits and boost your energy, so let's get started.

Stocking the Essentials

Setting a good foundation in your kitchen will help spur your success in adopting the pescatarian lifestyle. First, get prepared. Read this to learn about the essentials for optimal success. Second, take inventory of your current pantry, refrigerator, and freezer. You may have more than you think! Surveying your list will help you save money by avoiding duplicate purchases. This is also an excellent time to toss expired pantry items (or those with too much freezer burn). Organize your pantry using the "first in, first out" system to prevent waste in the future. Place items with a sooner expiration date closer to the front and those with a later date behind them. Next, eliminate what you don't need or use. Donate these items to a local food pantry. Finally, stock up to save time later. Head to the store to restock your pantry, refrigerator, and freezer with the necessities to succeed on a pescatarian plan.

The Pantry

Canned beans: Canned beans are among the most flexible and inexpensive plant-based proteins to stock in your pantry. Full of fiber, too, canned beans can be used in salads, soups, snacks, main dishes, and even desserts (you must try the Blender Black Bean Brownies).

Canned salmon: As an inexpensive alternative to fresh-caught salmon, canned salmon is packed with protein, omega-3 fatty acids, and even calcium (if it contains bones). For a fraction of the price, you can always eat the pescatarian way if you have canned salmon (and other fish, like sardines and tuna).

These tiny chia seeds are a nutritious superstar and versatile in the kitchen. Sprinkle them on any dish for an extra nutrient boost as they contain a balance of healthy fats, plant-based protein, and fiber. Plus, when added to liquid, chia seeds gel, absorbing up to nine times their weight in liquid and creating a pudding-like texture.

Diced canned tomatoes: Did you know that US-grown canned tomatoes go from farm to can within hours? This locks in their nutrients, including lycopene, vitamins C and E, and potassium, so you get the most out of this seasonal fruit. Plus, canned tomatoes contain more of the antioxidant lycopene than fresh vegetables, which helps reduce inflammation and ward off chronic diseases.

Dry whole-grains (farro, buckwheat, bulgur, quinoa, etc.): Whole-grains are a staple on the pescatarian diet because they're high in fiber, vitamins, and minerals. Replacing refined white grains with whole-grains will boost your heart health, improve blood sugar control, and more. There are more than 20 types of whole-grains to choose from, so have fun experimenting over time.

Quality oils: Not all oils are created equally. Opt for pure heart-healthy oils rich in monounsaturated fats, like olive oil and avocado oil. Avocado oil is the preferred option for higher cooking temperatures because of its higher smoke point, while olive oil is used in dressings and marinades; however, both can safely be used interchangeably.

Rolled oats: A deliciously nutritious breakfast staple, multipurpose oats are rich in fiber, B vitamins, magnesium, iron, and more, plus they're inexpensive.

Spices: A well-stocked spice rack is one of the easiest ways to enhance your meal's flavor without adding fat or calories. Many spices contain unique health benefits from warding off the common cold to easing digestive discomfort. If you're just building your spice cabinet, start with the basics—salt, pepper, garlic powder, oregano, cinnamon, red pepper flakes, smoked paprika, cumin, chili powder, and curry powder.

The Refrigerator

Avocados: Rich in healthy fats, fiber, and antioxidants, avocados are a "superfood" you should have on hand to mash on toast, add to smoothies, turn into sauces and dressings, throw in a salad, or use in burgers like the Tuna Avocado Burgers. When shopping finds, avocados that are soft to squeeze, but not mushy. If you remove the stem at the top, it should be green, not brown.

Eggs: Eggs are a quick, easy, and versatile protein source to stock in your refrigerator. When possible, look for the terms "organic," "free-range," and "no added hormones." Although "pasture-raised" is not a regulated term, these eggs have been found to contain more anti-inflammatory omega-3 fatty acids and vitamin D.

Fresh fish and shellfish: You'll learn how to select the best fish later in the, but always ask your fishmonger what's freshest when at the fish counter.

Fresh herbs: Add fresh herbs for a bright burst of flavor and plenty of health benefits. Parsley, cilantro, dill, rosemary, and thyme are just a few favorites featured throughout the recipes in this book.

Fruit: Most Americans do not consume the recommended two to three servings of fruit per day. Stock your refrigerator with your favorites, so you always have an easy snack option. Berries, apples, and pears contain the most fiber but also shop for melons, bananas, and stone fruits for variety.

Organic tofu: Tofu is an excellent source of plant-based protein and calcium, which is why it's perfect for the pescatarian diet. Organic tofu is inexpensive and GMO-free.

Vegetables: You can't go wrong when stocking your refrigerator with vegetables. When shopping, your cart should look like a rainbow.

The Freezer

Frozen fish: Frozen fish is an affordable way to incorporate seafood into your diet. Minimal nutrients, if any, are lost in the freezing process.

Frozen fruit: Frozen fruit is typically more affordable than fresh, and it's an excellent option for off-season fruit. It's picked and frozen at its peak ripeness, which also means its peak nutrient content.

Frozen vegetables: If you often let fresh vegetables spoil, opt for frozen! Picked, processed, and frozen at their peak ripeness, frozen plants are an excellent alternative to raw.

The Hardware

You don't need a Michelin-star-worthy kitchen to follow the pescatarian diet. Aside from an oven and stove, plus necessary kitchen utensils (like a spatula, spoon, and tongs), here are five kitchen essentials that will help you eat the pescatarian way:

Nesting mixing bowls: Whether you're making a salad, mixing cookie dough, or prepping vegetables to roast, a set of nesting mixing bowls will be helpful in your kitchen. If possible, find a game with matching lids for secure storage in your refrigerator.

For easy cleanup, parchment paper is a must-have in your pescatarian kitchen. Line sheet pans with parchment paper when roasting vegetables or baking fish to reduce cleaning time. Preparing fish en papillote, or in a pouch made from parchment paper, is a quick and straightforward technique.

Sauté pan or cast-iron pan: The best way to get crispy skin on fish is to pan-sear it on your stovetop. A heavy sauté pan or cast-iron pan is the best kitchen tool to use for this. Bonus points if your container is oven safe!

Sharp chef's knife: Investing in a good chef's knife, and knowing how to use it, will make prep time a breeze! A good knife has a sturdy cutting board that doesn't slide with each cut.

Sheet pans: Whether you're roasting, baking, or broiling, sheet pans are necessary to get the job done. Look for rimmed sheet pans to prevent spills in your oven.

13. Smart Spending

The pescatarian diet can cost a pretty penny since seafood is one of the most expensive proteins available. You can be a smart shopper and spend less, however, by following these tips:

1. Plan your meals to avoid waste. Making your own, you'll prevent food waste and buy only what you need and use for the week.

2. Choose frozen over fresh. Frozen seafood, vegetables, fruit, and even grains can be more affordable than their new counterparts. Much of the fish you see "fresh" at the fish counter was frozen (check the signs and ask your fishmonger). Even more, you don't have to worry about waste as much when buying frozen foods, since they last longer and don't have to be used right away.

3. Eat seasonally. In-season produce and fish are less expensive, so plan your meals accordingly. The crab season is in the fall and winter. Reserve your crab intake for these months to get the biggest bang for your buck!

4. Use a bulk frozen fish delivery service. Several frozen food delivery services allow you to purchase high-quality fish and shellfish in bulk at discounted prices. Frozen is just as nutritious as fresh, so don't be shy about using these services (if you have the freezer space).

5. Shop for staples online. Frequently, buying nonperishable staples, including dry grains, canned beans, canned tomatoes, canned fish, and oil online, can save you money. Just as you may price-compare your local supermarkets, shop around online between different vendors to find the best deals.

14. Selecting and Preparing Fish And Seafood

Is preparing fish and shellfish intimidating to you? You're not alone.

Maybe it's the scaly skin, hard shells, or googly eyes staring back at you. Perhaps it's fear of a fishy scent lingering throughout your home. Or maybe attempts resulted in a dry, overpriced home experiment that didn't turn out favorably. Whatever fishy beliefs you may have, purchasing, preparing, and cooking seafood are much easier than you think.

You don't have to worry about many of these common obstacles if you're just getting started. There are foolproof ways to master cooking fish at home.

First, choose a doable recipe. Instead of cooking a whole fish, try baking a flaky fish fillet, like the Slow-Roasted Dijon Arctic Char. In place of preparing mussels or clams, choose a more natural shellfish, like peeled and deveined shrimp, to boost your confidence. Get help at the fish counter. You don't need to fillet and debone your fish to be successful. Second, choose an affordable option to ease your fears of wasting money. Start with frozen or canned seafood to get your feet wet. Last, be sure to stay focused in the kitchen. Fish has a short cooking time, making it easy to go from flaky fillet to dry and overcooked quickly, but there's no need to be intimidated. Don't leave the kitchen while your fish cooks and avoid multitasking. As a guide, your fish is fully cooked when it becomes opaque and the flesh flakes when pressed with a fork.

And remember, if at first, you don't succeed, try and try again. There are so many fish varieties available; the fish counter is your oyster (pun intended)!

7.   PREPPING FOR THE KETOGENIC DIET

At this point, you are surely eager to get started with the Keto diet. Whether you have chosen to follow the SKD or any of the other types, you will find that making the most of your chosen approach. That is why this is focused on helping you get the most out of your new eating plan by keeping in mind some fundamental guidelines and recommendations.

 So, do take the time to go over this while considering the finer points of the Keto diet. You will surely find that making the most of your diet plan will help you achieve your goals in far less time than you might initially think it could take.

Importance of Nutrition on the Ketogenic Pescatarian Diet

The first part of success on the Ketogenic Pescatarian Diet is learning how to hone in on your nutrition. As we have throughout this book, the Ketogenic Pescatarian Diet is a low-carb, moderate-protein, high-fat diet. While there are many moving parts to this diet, it is essential that you master the basics before you try to get fancy with your results. Following the basic rules of the food, you will find you are going to start losing weight like you never thought was possible.

As a regular woman, losing weight might seem like an uphill battle. Later in this book, you will find delicious recipes to help fuel your health instead of harming it. Through nutrition alone, you will be able to improve your health but paired with a proper exercise program, and you will reach those results even quicker!

Remember that before you begin your diet, it is going to be vital that you find your macronutrients to help you reach your goals. If you are genuinely looking for life-changing results, these numbers cannot just be guessed.

Getting your body into ketosis takes a proper science. As you will recall from the first book, we all have a different carbohydrate limit. When you find your limit, you will discover how easy or hard it will be for you to get into ketosis.

Importance of Exercise on Ketogenic Pescatarian Diet

At this moment, you probably already realize that diet and exercise is essential for your health. While this is true, the combination of the two is going to be a bit more complicated than that while following the ketogenic diet. For this reason, you will have to be a bit more mindful about your new lifestyle, especially if you are just starting on the Ketogenic Diet.

When you begin restricting carbs in your diet, this is going to cause a chain-reaction of changes within your body. Some of these changes that occur may affect your performance when it comes to exercise; this is why it is going to be so crucial that you are cautious with your choices. You see, by restricting carbohydrates, you will be limiting your muscle cells from access to sugar as per usual. When your cells are lacking this sugar, your muscles will no longer be able to function at high intensities.

For this reason, athletes are typically on a less-strict version of the Ketogenic Diet. If you are looking to lose weight, the good news is that you will be able to do this with diet alone. By incorporating exercise, you will be able to maximize your results without needing crazy exercise routines.

The key to success here is going to be finding your perfect macronutrients to fuel your exercise routines. As you can see, these two elements of a healthier lifestyle are going to go hand in hand!

Before You Begin the Ketogenic Pescatarian Diet

Before you begin your diet, I invite you to take a few moments to think about your why. WHY are you looking to change your life? Are you improving your experience for yourself? Is it for your children? Your Grandchildren? We all have a different reason as to why we want to become healthier. I want you to use your why to fuel your success while following the Ketogenic Diet.

Remember that for anyone, weight loss is going to be a prolonged process. This is why it is so easy for people to give up before they reach their goal. Every time you think about giving up or cheating on your diet, think about your why and get right back on track.

Before you begin planning for your diet, try to set yourself up for success. The very first step is going to be setting realistic goals for yourself. If you give yourself an unattainable goal, you are already setting yourself up for failure. As you select your personal goals for your diet, focus on small benchmarks. An example of this would be to eat one good meal in a day or lose five pounds in the first month. When you hit your goals because they are attainable, this gives you a burst of confidence to keep going!

With that in mind, remember that there is no reason for you to change your lifestyle overnight! Up until this point, you have probably lived your life in a very particular way. While this may not be what is best for you, nobody is expecting you to blow up your metabolism and just be healthier all of a sudden! You will raise your chances of success by taking the race slow and steady. Even if you just start by lowering your calorie intake by 200 calories, you will still lose weight! By making it slow, you will avoid burning yourself out.

Speaking of burning yourself out, remember that there is no reason to be a perfectionist on your new diet. You are going to experience some setbacks! Remember that your body is going to go through some significant changes. When you think about it, it is pretty amazing you can run off of fat instead of glucose in the first place. As you go through the process, remember to be kind to yourself, and when you experience a setback, take a breath, and keep going!

For some, your motivation may be enough for you, but if not, it is always an excellent idea to find a buddy to experience this with! You may be surprised how many people out there have similar goals to yours. It is essential to have a support group while following the new diet to call on for motivation and a boost in your willpower. This way, when you hit one of those speedbumps or are suffering through the keto flu, you have someone to go through it with. When you are in something together, you will end up on the other side as more energetic individuals.

Finally, remember to be patient and reward yourself for all of the excellent work you are putting into yourself. When you think about it, the weight you have now didn't just happen overnight. Your weight loss is going to take a while, too, but the important part is that you are doing something about it!

The truth is, dieting is hard work for everyone, and sometimes, it just isn't any fun! A way to keep yourself going through the tough times is to give yourself a small reward! As you set your mini-goals for your weight loss, reward yourself with mini bonuses! Whether you reward yourself with a bubble bath, a new pair of pants, or a great massage, celebrate the small things!

At this point, I hope you are feeling motivated and excited to begin your new journey on the Ketogenic Diet. It is going to take work, and it is going to be hard at times, but you can get through anything! Once you get the basics down and get into a routine, the only thing you will be asking yourself is, why didn't you start sooner!

Remember that at the end of this book, you will be provided with meal plans and exercise routines. While they are just suggestions, they will stand as a great building block for you. Eventually, you will be able to write your plans based on your personal goals.

Set your goals in writing

When you write down your goals, you are making a written contract with yourself. This written contract will allow you to keep yourself accountable to… well, yourself. You don't need to be responsible for anyone else. You know who you are, what you want, and where you want to be. That is why it is of the utmost importance for you to become aware of what you need to accomplish.

With that in mind, some folks find it useful to keep a journal. It doesn't have to be much. It could even be an excel spreadsheet with dates and ideas. In this journal, you can keep track of what you are doing and your achievements. So, if you are looking to lose weight, you can track your influence. If you are looking to improve your stamina, you can keep track of your workouts. Or, if you are looking to improve health, you can keep track of the medication you are taking. You might be surprised to find that your doctor may even begin to cut back on your meds.

But all of this begins with your ability to stay on track. To do so, you need to have a clear picture of what your goals look like. After all, how far would you get if you hopped in your car and just drove? You might not get very now. But if you are clear on where you are going, even if it will take you days to reach your destination, you will eventually get there.

Reaching your ultimate goal is a matter of focus and dedication. This is not a sprint. This is more like a marathon. And as any marathon runner will tell you, you need to pace yourself. By walking yourself, you will eventually get to where you want to be. You might not be in the first place, but just the satisfaction of finishing the race might make it seem like you were the winner.

8.   MISTAKES TO AVOID ON A KETOGENIC DIET

I need to cover some of the mistakes that I frequently see humans make on a ketogenic food regimen. If you can keep away from those errors, you will be much more likely to shed pounds and feel better.

15. Mistake #1: Bad Mindset

Many human beings deal with the Ketogenic Pescatarian Diet as something they'll "attempt for a week or two."

They want to dip their toe within the water to look if the weight loss program "works." But they don't want to commit.

There are two problems with this technique. If you're no longer committed, then you are going to give up at the first signal of hassle. If you get tempted or do not lose weight for some days, you may give it all up. And I can assure you that now not the entirety will move flawlessly for you. It by no means does.

The second hassle is that no weight loss program works except your technique as a lifestyle.

If you need, you could lose a few weights after which pass again to ingesting bread, pasta, and sugar. But in case you move back to consuming the one's ingredients, you'll also give lower back to gaining weight. That is what we name the yo-yo dieting trap.

16. Mistake #2: Eating Too Much

Many people have developed bad eating habits. We'll consume until the whole thing is long past on our plates, we're going to devour when it is mealtime as opposed to when we're hungry. And we're going to snack all day instead of consuming actual meals.

All of this, unfortunately, leads to a variety of overeating.

17. Mistake #3: Not Testing

Our bodies are all a bit one-of-a-kind. Two human beings eating the equal Ketogenic Pescatarian Diet can now and again get specific results.

One man or woman could be in ketosis and dropping weight, and another character could be struggling.

That's why testing is so important. You want to ensure that you're without a doubt in ketosis. And if you aren't, then you could make modifications to your weight loss program and life.

When you're in ketosis, your frame will produce ketone our bodies. There are three varieties of ketone our bodies: Acetoacetate (AcAc), Beta-hydroxybutyrate (BHB), and Acetone.

In your blood, you may degree all three ketones our bodies. In your urine, AcAc and Acetone can be measured. And for your breath, simply Acetone.

Your blood ketone degrees are an excellent indicator of ketosis. Unfortunately, measuring blood ketone levels is also the most high-priced method.

That's why many humans still degree their urine and breath ketone ranges alternatively.

For weight loss, you don't need to chase high ketone ranges measuring and tracking ketones is just another way to get more records about what's occurring for your body, so do not get caught on ketone levels!

18. Mistake #4: Not Eating Enough Nutrient-Dense Foods

On a ketogenic weight loss plan, you'll pay several attentions to the macronutrients you devour, and you can use our Keto Calculator to figure out the right share of fats, carbs, and protein for you: keto summit keto-calculator

But consider that you also need to be getting enough nutrients and minerals.

You might be aware of some terrible matters that happen in case you're critically deficient in a micronutrient. For example,

You can get scurvy in case you don't get sufficient vitamin C.

You can get goiter if you're deficient in iodine.

Or you could cross blind in case you don't get sufficient diet A.

Another amazing test to take into account is a DEXA scan. This test will degree your fats ranges in addition to your bone and muscle degrees. If you do it before you begin your food plan, you will be able to music later, precisely how properly your food plan is working.

Besides those acute issues, continual deficiencies also can be a huge hassle. Often, nutrient deficiencies are not so severe which you exhibit a specific disease. That doesn't mean, though, that they may be not making you less healthy.

Over time, if you're low in nutrients and minerals, your frame just may not feature well. That can result in illnesses, fatigue, and more significant. Even minor nutrition and mineral deficiencies are probably making it more robust so one can shed pounds.

A smooth manner to enhance your micronutrient intake is to consume more nutrient-dense ingredients. Most of those foods in shape nicely right into a ketogenic eating regimen. For instance, inexperienced leafy vegetables, organ meats, and seafood are all ketogenic-friendly. And they maybe some of the most nutrient-dense meals you could devour.

Supplementation with a terrific multivitamin or veggies powder is likewise helpful.

If you're into checking out, then attempt getting a SpectraCell evaluation, or a Urine Organic Acid take a look at. Both of these assessments will tell you which vitamins and minerals you are deficient in. That way,you can focus mainly on those deficiencies.

19. Mistake #5: Eating Toxic, Inflammatory Foods - Even if They're Low Carb

Not everything low in carbs is right for you. Period.

For example, you can go to maximum grocery stores these days and discover low-carb processed ingredients. You can get low-carb bread, low-carb cookies, and low-carb snacks.

You might be capable of stay in ketosis while consuming the one's low-carb foods, but they may be nonetheless awful for your body. Many of them contain wheat, gluten, and different inflammatory components.

And as I mentioned, the inflammation usually makes it more difficult for you to shed pounds.

Here are components that I recommend avoiding, even in low-carb meals:

Wheat, Rye, and Barley. The new era has created a manner to make these foods low-carb on occasion. But they nevertheless always include gluten, so   one can inevitably motive irritation to   your frame.   Plus, they are not very nutrient-dense.

Dairy. Yes even cheese. In summary, dairy is probably ok. The hassle is which you do not live in an abstract world. Milk will pretty much always hold you out of ketosis. And the vast majority of humans have some degree of sensitivity to dairy products like cheese. (This is maximum probably actual even in case you are not lactose-intolerant.) Plus, you are in all likelihood to overeat cheese and cream!

Vegetable and Seed Oils. This includes Vegetable Oil, Canola Oil, Corn Oil, Sunflower Oil, and similar merchandise. Your cooking oil also makes a significant distinction in your weight loss. As Dr. Shanahan points out in her book, Deep Nutrition, those oils produce trans-fats, which can block your enzymes for burning fats.

Any food you have an intolerance to. Start paying greater interest to your body. If you wake up sooner or later and notice which you're congested or that your joints are stiff, ask yourself what you ate. You're possibly touchy to one of the meals you ate the day earlier than.

Also, be careful with nuts. Many people have allergies or sensitivities to nuts. But extra than that, nuts are easy to overeat. A ketogenic weight-reduction plan is not magic, so consuming 3,000 energy of nuts in step with day goes to make a difference.

20. Mistake #6: Ignoring Sleep, Exercise, and Stress

While ingesting a proper diet is essential for weight loss, it's not all that matters. Much weight-loss research has pressured the importance of sleep (7+ hours), exercise, and destressing. It's tough to get everything proper all at once.

Still, any small efforts you make in those areas can pay off inside the end.

21. Mistake #7: Not Being Patient

So if you're going to give the ketogenic eating regimen a strive, then simply supply it a try to be patient.

It's taken you a lifetime of eating poorly to get to where you're at. You can't assume to repair all that harm in only a few weeks.

22. Mistake #8: Not Eating Enough Fiber

Mainstream vitamins have gotten a lot of things wrong.

The importance of fiber is not one of them. The past few years of scientific research have shown simply how crucial thread is for your intestine health.

In particular, soluble fiber and resistant starches from veggies can enhance your gut bacteria. Fermented ingredients like sauerkraut are additionally exquisite in this regard.

And in case you have problem-consuming enough veggies, then take a tremendous prebiotic like the CoBionic Foundation.

9.   WEIGHT LOSS AND EXERCISE

We all know that exercise is right for you and that it can help you lose weight, but we don't necessarily do it. Many individuals are giving the excuse that they don't want to be huge and bulky or don't have enough time; the truth isn't many people like to exercise and get bored. You will learn a simple workout that you can do in no time; thus, you won't have any excuse to practice anymore. Exercise keeps you healthy, glad, and enables you to sleep much more accessible.

Contrary to the common faith, working out on days of fasting can effectively lead to a higher level of muscle building and fat burning than working out on average days. Noradrenaline concentrations are higher when fasting, enabling you to practice harder while increasing the attention of human growth hormones assist in boosting muscle mass. Misinformed and uninformed individuals indicate that fasting lowers muscle mass, which is not a fact.

If you want to burn fat by following any diet or regiment, one fact that remains constant is that you have to take fewer calories than you burn. You need to generate a calorie deficit of that quantity to lose a certain amount. You can't locate a fat-burning post or book and forget the term ' calories,' so what are they? These are food's energy. Calories power every action in your body, so your body needs them always.

Calories are obtained from carbohydrates, fats, and proteins and are your body's primary source of energy. They are either used as physical energy or deposited as body fat regardless of where they came from. Stored calories will remain as fat in your body unless used up by reducing the intake of calories so that your body can use up the reserves or burn more calories than you take in by physical exercise. It's excellent for you to exercise and make you feel good.

How do you calculate the calories you eat, the calories you need to burn, and the calories you burned during your workout? Check the nutritional content of the food supplied on the back or side of the box to calculate the calories in the food you bought from the store. There are distinct quantities of calories per unit in each macronutrient. Twenty grams of protein include four calories, 35 grams of carbohydrate contains four calories, and 15 grams of fat add nine calories. Calculate the food's calorific value by multiplying the caloric equal of each macronutrient. These nutrients are always calculated in grams. To discover the complete calories of the meals, add the calories provided off by each macronutrient. When calculating the number of calories like this, you will not only find out the calorific value but also incorporate it into a balanced diet. The serving size and the number of servings contained must be taken into account. Nearly all of them indicate only one serving's calorific amount, the number of meals can alter the calorie count. Always compare the number of nutrients you are taking with the recommended values, so you don't eat too much or too little. Online calculators and guide books can also be used to help you do this.

You should first know your basal metabolic rate to know how many calories you burn during the workout session. This is the amount of energy that your body uses to work. There is no constant number because everything depends on several factors. Age is one of the determining factors for your BMR. The older you are, the lower your BMR, the more exercise you will need. A muscular person is more likely to burn more fat than a fat person. The ambient temperature also serves apart as the higher your BMR will be. The hotter it is, the higher your BMR is this because you are warmed up by the setting, so more calories are invested in losing weight. Work out duration is also a significant factor, the better, the longer, but don't overdo it. The fitter you are, the fewer calories you will consume as your body is already used to it. Your diet has a direct effect on your metabolism. If you don't consume enough, drink too much, or exercise any other poor dietary habits, your metabolism will be impacted, thus decreasing the number of calories you burn. Lack of sufficient sleep can cause you to consume more calories as you become more exhausted, and practice is more probable, but it can also impact your metabolism. Oxygen helps to offer energy to your body to continue to work. You will consume more calories if you breathe more strongly during workouts.

Some conventional methods are available to approximate the number of calories you burn in a day. Everyone has their strengths and weaknesses, so it's best to use them all and use the mean as the estimate for the best results. The first is by using exercise devices such as the Fit bit to monitor your regular motions and assess calories consumed during the period they are held. While it has been discovered that the number of calories burned is not entirely precise, they are convenient and straightforward. Metabolic screening is another technique. The machinery needed for this technique in laboratories and clinics can be accessed affordably from there as they are costly. These examinations can assist you in changing what you eat and your exercise regiment, but some individuals do not think the price of this technique is worth it. Always try to ensure that a skilled technician tests you so you can get the most accurate results. The last but mostly used is online calculators. These calculators are trying to offer your weekly spending an estimated value. The amount they offer is very general, but they can be used as your weight loss guideline. Calculating the mean of all these techniques will provide you with a near assessment of how many calories you consume in a day.

Yes, exercising on an empty stomach is okay and secure. A generally healthy adult can usually practice on an empty stomach without having any adverse reactions. Working out without eating will result in you burning more body fat. You are more likely to have more energy when you're in a fasted state to do your workout routine.

However, if you have experienced fainting, feeling dizzy, or weak after practice during a fasted state, do not continue doing it. Always listen to your body; without even knowing it, you might destroy it. By organizing an exercise timetable that operates well with your fasting timetable as you can organize your time table in any direction you like, you can manage around this. Fasted exercise can speed up the weight loss process.

There is a fat-burning myth that you have to eat fat to lose body fat when you exercise. At first, it may seem embarrassing why discovering reality is not real but read on. People believe that when carrying out an aerobic workout that encourages peak fat loss, there is a particular sweet spot. During low-intensity practice, a higher quantity of fat is used, but the entire amount of fat used is low. Increasing exercise intensity improves the amount of fat used.

The impacts of various intensities of aerobic exercise have been likened, and the typical finding is that the total fat loss is equivalent regardless of the strength at which the practice was performed, provided the caloric consumption is the same. This implies that the quantity of calories used during training is more essential than the energy used. The body decreases fat as soon as it burns more calories than it eats. Exercise intensity and length are inversely proportional. The higher the concentration of activity requires, the lower the workout length. For a lengthy period of high-intensity exercise for a brief period, you can attempt a low-intensity task to fit your body best.

If you want a healthy heart and lungs, you should look after your body. Strength training is essential. There's no doubt that organizations make you feel beautiful, and they also help you burn calories while you're sleeping. If you enhance your muscle amount, your sensitivity to insulin will also increase. To help boost your muscle mass, you should develop a fitness exercise scheme to reduce your weight and improve muscle mass.

During aerobic exercise, the calorie expenditure is average, five calories/minute during a low-intensity workout, and around ten calories/minute during a high-intensity workout. Two exercise days, even if you burn more calories, do not equal the fat-burning of losing calories across several days. You should exercise like three times/week, but the division between weights, interval training, and weights depends on your goals.

If you do exercise, but you do not change your diet, your weight loss process will be prolonged. It is not easy to reach a point that the amount of fat you will burn will be directly proportional to the amount and time you spend exercising. About nine calories/minute are used during weight training. On top of burning calories through exercise, there are also more calories lost after the practice, which is called excess post-exercise oxygen consumption. It is due to an increase in adrenalin and noradrenalin on top of other factors that make your system burn calories even after exercise from the fat stores. The magnitude of the post-exercise calorie loss is dependent on the intensity and duration in which the activity was carried out. Not many people can be able to sustain energy to the point that they generate a large EPOC.

Dieting without exercise is a common approach people undertake. The problem with it is that it leads to a loss in lean body mass and reduced metabolic rate. To make up for the calorie restriction, the system lowers the metabolic rate. As a result, your body can enter starvation mode; thus, you will not lose weight. When food intake is returned, the lowered metabolism results in regain of the fat that was lost. It is not an effective long term plan. If you eat too little and exercise more, you may enter into starvation mode, which can stop fat loss completely. Achieving the equilibrium between exercise and dietary alterations to enhance weight loss while preventing muscle loss is the ultimate goal. Getting more muscular will raise your metabolic rate.

High-interval intensity training, HIIT, is an exercise method that works incredibly with to promote weight loss and results in more significant weight loss than lower intensity continuous workout. You simply switch between periods of high-intensity activity and periods of low-intensity exercise. The practice can suit your timetable, however tight your schedule is. It allows you in a short time to get the advantages of lengthy workout sessions. There are different kinds of intermittent fasting you can attempt. If you like cycling, you could: warm-up with soft cycling, start pedaling after a minute as you do and boost the strength, after 15 seconds your bodies get tired, if you can proceed at the same speed then the power you set is not big enough, you will discover your ideal fierce resistance after practicing severely after fast-cycling reduces the strength. By walking, swimming, and any other workout that can be performed quickly, you can also do HIIT without a bicycle.

10.   STRICT DIET FOR FAT BURNING

23. Eat More Cruciferous Vegetables

Incorporate more cruciferous veggies like broccoli and cauliflower in your diet. This group of vegetables is known as the crucifers, in light of the flowers that often sprout looking like a cross. They contain an assortment of healthy mixes, including sulforaphane, founded by Dr. Paul Talley, M.D., at Johns Hopkins University. Talley distinguished this specific compound in broccoli, taxi bagel, watercress, and other cruciferous vegetables as having the best ability to deliver detoxifying proteins. He later found that broccoli sprouts, which appear as though horse feed sprouts, however, are not as thready, have ten to one hundred times more sulforaphane than broccoli does.

Cruciferous vegetables incorporate the following:

Arugula Bok choy Broccoli Broccolini

Broccoli rabe Broccoli sprouts

Brussels sprouts Cabbage Cauliflower Chinese cabbage Collard greens Kale

Mustard greens Rutabaga

Swiss chard Turnip greens Turnips Watercress

Sulforaphane, a cell reinforcement, accelerates the detoxification of numerous conceivably unsafe synthetic compounds, upgrades glutathione production, and is accepted to forestall malignant growth and stifle tumor development.

Another compound in crucifers called indole carbinol has been found to build the detoxification of estrogen in the liver by as much as 50 percent. This makes it incredibly gainful during weight loss when the liver is immersed with estrogen-like synthetics from fat stores. Indole carbinol is also accepted to battle disease, particularly bosom and prostate malignant growth.

How to Do It: Aim for in any event two servings of cruciferous vegetables per day (1 serving = 1/2 cup cooked, 1 cup crude, or 1/4 cup broccoli sprouts). One route is to add arugula to your serving of mixed greens. While the more significant part of us consider arugula an option in contrast to lettuce, it's a cruciferous vegetable. It contains more vitamin C and calcium than some other plate of mixed greens green, along with folic acid and other vitamins and minerals. On the off chance that you locate arugula's impactful, peppery bite to be a bit overpowering, search for child arugula, which is less spicy and hot, or have a go at blending it in with other serving of mixed greens to soften the taste. Arugula servings of mixed greens taste good with dressings made with lemon juice, balsamic vinegar, extra virgin olive oil, or hazelnut oil.

Another option is cauliflower, one of the couples of cruciferous vegetables (along with turnips) that can be utilized as a substitute for boring foods. Take a stab at hacking it finely in the food processor to reenactor the surface of the rice, or squashing it—a more beneficial option as it contains about 33% of the calories of potatoes. Attempt the flavorful Chicken Stir-fry over the "Rice" formula in this book, which utilizes cauliflower rather than rice. My favorite method to eat cauliflower is as a snack. I slash it into bitesize pieces, hurl it with extra virgin olive oil and a bit of ocean salt, and meal it in the grill until it's gently caramelized. You can include cumin, cayenne, or other flavors since enormous quantities can debilitate thyroid function. Any cooking, whether it's steaming, bubbling, heating, broiling, barbecuing, or microwaving, deactivates the undesirable thyroid impeding mixes.

Eat-in Color

The shade of each fruit and vegetable offers more than aesthetic intrigue. We can categorize a plant's specific nutritional worth dependent on its color, which is brought about by phytonutrients or plant supplements. Each color sneaks up suddenly as far as your body's ability to get more fit.

The Purple Protectors (Purple or Red)

This gathering contains anthocyanins (pronounced a homomer union), water-soluble cell reinforcements that diminish the danger of malignant growth, coronary illness, diabetes, and hypersensitivities, and forestall DNA harm, inflammation, and untimely maturing. A vital piece of the diet, this gathering has the following explicit benefits:

Has characteristic calming properties that improve insulin and leptin sensitivity

Strengthens veins and vessels, decreasing varicose veins and cellulite formation

Helps forestall obesity

Is high in fiber (particularly raspberries)

Reduces the breakdown of collagen by inflammatory synthetic concoctions, which anticipates skin maturing

Beets Blackberries Black Currants Blueberries Cherries Cranberries Eggplant Plums Pomegranates Purple cabbage Raspberries Red apple Strawberries

Beets are stacked with betaine, a liver securing cancer prevention agent that has been found to help the liver procedure fats and keep fat from accumulating in the liver. In one investigation, betaine supplements fundamentally improved liver catalysts and diminished fat deposits in the liver. Creature concentrates also show that betaine can improve liver function and secure against chemical harm to the liver.

Blueberries are one of the highest in cell reinforcements of any fruit or vegetable. They contain the phytochemical anthocyanidins and are wealthy in gelatin, the fiber that ties to poisons and also helps lower cholesterol. Blueberries also have a compound like cranberries, called epic ate jawline, and can be utilized to forestall urinary tract infections.

Raspberries, strawberries, and pomegranates contain ellagic corrosive and intensify that has been found to secure against liver harm, improve glutathione, kill poisons, and diminish the weight impacts of endocrine disruptors.

Raspberries are especially useful for you. As of late, Japanese scientists isolated a compound in raspberries that has one of a kind weightless impact. They gave creatures a high-fat diet for ten weeks. They found that supplementing the menu with the raspberry compound diminished stomach fat, triglycerides, all-out muscle to fat ratio, and by and substantial weight, and improved their ability to consume fat.

24. How to Do It:

Each day, eat at any rate one serving (1 serving = 3/4 cup) of the purple protectors, whether it includes a handful of new or solidified berries to your morning meal, getting a charge out of straightforward, however delightful sweet!

Have a go at having beets with supper. Beets can be bubbled, pureed, roasted, flame-broiled, or cured. Bubble them unpeeled and leave an inch of the green stem in any event, so the color doesn't drain. Raw beets can be ground into plates of mixed greens or squeezed with other vegetables. Opportunity to cook them, search for canned beets at the market. Keep away from jostled beets, which as a rule, accompany included sugar. Beets have a hearty sweetness that is best supplemented in plates of mixed greens by vinaigrette with lemon, apple juice vinegar, or balsamic vinegar, and intense flavors, for example, arugula, olives, and feta cheddar.

If you are in a hurry, attempt unsweetened pomegranate juice, which has a dark red color and a tart taste, Blueberry juice is another option. You can drink the milk, or have a go at blending 1/4 cup of pomegranate squeezes in with a solitary serving of nonfat organic vanilla yogurt in a bowl for a snappy smoothie. Even though you lose the fiber by drinking rather than eating these fruits, you'll despite everything appreciate the other medical advantages of eating these purple protectors.

The Extraordinary Oranges (Yellow, Orange, or Green)

This is the biggest gathering, containing fat-soluble phytonutrients called carotenoids (pronounced vehicle rotenoids). As the name infers, these plant shades give carrots their orange color. This gathering includes vegetables and fruits running from yellow to green to orange because the green pigmented chlorophyll that provides plants with their trademark green color can dominate the orange shade in specific foods.

Beta-carotene is the most popular carotenoid. However, this gathering also incorporates other carotenoids, for example, lutein (pronounced Lehigh schooler), lycopene, alpha-carotene, and foods plentiful in vitamin C and the related bioflavonoids. The following vegetables and fruits contain carotenoids:

Vegetables Fruit

Ringer peppers Carrots Green beans Leafy greens Lettuce Peas, green Peppers Pumpkin Spinach Squash Sweet Potatoes Tomatoes Zucchini Apricots Cantaloupes

Clementine's Grapefruit, pink Guava Honeydew Kiwi Lemons Nectarines Oranges Passionfruit Peaches Pears Persimmons Tangerines Watermelon The amazing oranges do an assortment of essential functions required for weight loss.

They ensure our phone films (which are made out of more than 30 percent fat) and other tissues from poison harm during weight loss.

They improve the sensitivity of insulin.

In specific, lycopene, a carotenoid found in tomatoes, decreases the danger of cardiovascular infection.

The orange gathering also contains foods high in vitamin C, which is essential during weight loss for the following reasons:

Aids in the formation of the appetite suppress neurotransmitters serotonin and dopamine

Helps forestall pressure-related weight gain in the guts

Boosts glutathione levels and is associated with deactivating poisons

Reduces inflammation by affecting histamine discharge and degradation

It lowers the measure of cholesterol in bile by converting cholesterol to bile acids, making bile more averse to bunch together and forming stones.

Watermelon, red chime peppers, melon, and kiwi. Be that as it may, my top pick for vitamin C is guava. However, harder to discover in the supermarket than other fruits, guava, a yellowish-green tropical fruit, rates high in vitamin C. Search for guava in Asian markets and some supermarkets. Maintain a strategic distance from guava juice, which is sweetened.

How to Do It: Include in any event two servings (1/2 cup every one) of the fantastic oranges consistently. Have a go at including diced ringer peppers or solidified slashed spinach to a morning meal omelet, pressing grape or cherry tomatoes to have with lunch, or microwaving solidified peas, green beans, or a little sweet potato to have with your supper rather than a white potato. If you, as a rule, have a plate of mixed greens, have a go at grinding raw carrots into the serving of mixed greens and substituting spinach rather than lettuce.

Numerous individuals who appreciate cooking with garlic and onions, remembering more of these foods for your diet ought to be simple. The dynamic phytonutrient in this family, called allicin, has been shown to lower cholesterol and pulse, forestall malignant growth, and improve general wellbeing. Here are only a couple of the weightless and medical advantages of this flavorful gathering:

Lowers absolute cholesterol, increments healthy HDL cholesterol, and forestalls the unsafe oxidation of LDL cholesterol

Improves detoxification by expanding the production of glutathione, allowing for the powerful elimination of poisons and carcinogenic substances

Foods in this gathering are:

Chives Endives

Garlic Leeks

Onions Scallions

Shallots

How to Do It: Aim for at any rate one serving of the correct whites every day (1 serving = 1/4 cup or one clove of garlic). Onions, garlic, shallots, chives, and scallions upgrade the flavor of various foods. If the idea of eating raw garlic causes you to wince, start with one clove, which despite everything, gives you a good measure of allicin (in any event 10 mg); however, generally doesn't bring about a perceivable garlic door. It should be squashed or hacked and added to food to discharge the allicin, rather than eaten entirety.

11. REACHING YOUR GOAL

The saying remains true — you will realize that what you put into your body is going to dictate how you feel. While on the Keto diet, you are building up energy stores for your body to utilize. This means that you should be feeling a necessary boost in your energy levels and the ability to get through each moment of each day without struggling. You can say goodbye to the sluggish feeling that often accompanies other diet plans. When you are on Keto, you should only be experiencing additional energy and unlimited potential. Your diet isn't going to always feel like a diet. After some time, you will realize that you enjoy eating a Keto menu very much. Because your body will be switching the way it metabolizes, it will also be switching what it craves. Don't be surprised if you end up craving fats and proteins as you progress on the Keto diet — this is what your body will eventually want.

Tracking Progress

Using a compare and contrast method is always great for tracking progress. Remember how you felt before starting the Keto diet. If you haven't started already, you can use this time to document your current state of being. Make sure to record your mindset and the cravings that you have. You can also mark down your current weight and BMI. When you have these figures to compare your progress to, you will be able to use this as a motivating tool. Remember to allow yourself to feel proud as you make it through each day of being on the Keto diet. Commit yourself and food. This will present its own set of challenges to face, but it is not going to be so complicated that you lose your way. Believe in your ability to see this through.

You Are What You Eat

Think about how you used to feel while eating your sugary and carb-loaded cravings. Your immediate response is likely going to suggest that you felt great but think about the bigger picture. Did you gain more energy from eating these things? Did you experience a crash after you ate them? Instant gratification might feel great at first, but you will likely have to deal with the consequences. Eating junk food only serves your immediate cravings. It also gets your body used to desire these things by reinforcing the behavior. Junk food holds no nutritional value, and it won't make you burn calories or use the sugar as a valid energy supply. When you think about it, this junk food indeed doesn't have a place in your life.

Know that you can obtain happiness in other ways that don't involve eating food. While eating does tend to be a social delight, it isn't the only thing that can make you happy when it comes to food. Choose to feel satisfied when you can know for sure that you are treating your body correctly. You should be able to handle the joy that comes from the fact that you are giving your body fuel that it can utilize. While eating your Keto-friendly food might not give you the same immediate rush eating your favorite junk food, it will benefit you much more in the long run. You will be able to notice its benefits long after you digest the food, and that is what is essential. A simple change in perspective is what you need to realize that your happiness isn't directly tied to the cravings that you satisfy. Your satisfaction needs to stem from a deeper place.

Eating tends to be an act of comfort when you are feeling down or worried. This is a cultural norm that many people experience. While being on the Keto diet, you will learn how to manage your emotions in a way that is not directly tied to the food you are eating. Instead of giving in to your cravings when you are having a hard day, the Keto diet teaches you to nourish yourself. When you are adequately fed, you will be able to boost your energy levels and maintain your endorphins.

As you know, this will be enough to give you some extra happiness when you need it. It is a more permanent solution to your problems that tend to linger. When you can think about things from this perspective, it will be easier to remember why you are on the Keto diet.

No diet should make you feel so miserable that you can't even enjoy its benefits. Keto is not a diet that should make you feel like you have no options. While on Keto, you should have the exact opposite experience. Because what you have to get rid of is minimal, you should be equipped with many different meals that you can enjoy on a guilt-free level. Diets that torment you emotionally are not suitable for you, no matter how healthy you are eating. With a healthy mind is just as important as having a healthy body. When your mindset begins to deteriorate, this will lessen your overall happiness levels. You are allowed to be happy while being on a diet! If you start to feel down, then something isn't right.

Through your example, other people will begin to see that Keto isn't as strict or complicated as they once thought. Being able to provide others with a real perspective can do a lot to keep the diet realistic. You can serve as an inspiration to your friends and loved ones to stick with your diet and remain happy and fulfilled. You may have likely tried to fake this feeling while being on nutrition in the past, but Keto does not involve any pretending. It is essential to listen to exactly how you are feeling and identify what makes you think this way. If you begin to experience anything negative, you are encouraged to alter your diet until you start to feel better. There should be no suffering while on the Keto diet!

Your Life Will Improve

There comes the point while being on the Keto diet that you make a shift from trying to succeeding. This will happen at various locations for people, but when it happens to you, embrace it. Instead of focusing on the fact that you are following a diet, you can begin to focus on the benefits you are receiving. You need to make sure that you are enjoying your life! There are so many things in life that try to get you down, so when you find something that brings you up, you should focus your attention on these things. One of the very first things that the Keto diet will provide you with is energy. As you have read, this is one of the benefits that you should experience reasonably quickly. Use your power to the best of your ability. Try to divide your time wisely, keeping in mind that the diet has allowed you some additional fuel to use throughout your day.

Even if you feel that your energy levels are currently on the rise, try to still practice healthy habits like going to bed earlier and waking up earlier. This is going to regulate your bodily systems further. What you need to remember is that the Keto diet is going to give you momentum. It is up to you to keep up with it. If you do nothing with it, then it is almost like these benefits are being wasted. When you can remain aware of them, you should be able to take full advantage of them. Try to practice as many healthy habits as you can when you first start noticing these new changes. This can be an exciting and uplifting time for you!

12. ADVANTAGES AND DISADVANTAGES OF KETOGENIC DIET

25. Advantages of Keto Diet

The keto diet may have several positive effects on the body. One of the most prominent positive aspects of the keto diet is the ease of sticking to the food. Successful weight loss plans must be easy to follow for most people to be successful. A low-carb diet may be easy to follow because the keto diet can significantly reduce appetite. If you don't feel hungry, you're more likely to stay on the diet plan. When a person consumes carbohydrates, there is a burst of energy and a feeling of fullness. Unfortunately, these sensations are short-lived because the glucose used to generate energy burns away quickly. This leads to hunger within a short period. While on keto, the fats will keep you feeling full for a more extended period. Additionally, as long as you are snacking on items within the plan, there is much room for high-fat items in the diet.

Another good thing about the keto diet, especially in the beginning, you will lose weight. By staying on the plan and following the tenets, you're likely to lose up to twice as much weight at the beginning of a diet as you will with low-fat, low-calorie foods. This is especially true during the first two or three weeks on the menu as the body sheds excess water.

The keto diet reduces the amount of fat stored in the body. The fat loss is made up of visceral fat. Visceral fat is fat that accumulates in the abdomen and tends to attach itself to organs. The keto diet may reduce fat, which is known to be the most harmful and may reduce the risk of heart disease and type 2 diabetes. These issues are often seen in people who are obese or only overweight. The visceral fat loss reduces the fat in the most dangerous areas of the body and improves overall health in many individuals.

Ketogenic diets allow you to shed off extra weight without risking diseases rapidly. The Ketogenic Pescatarian Diet restricts the intake of carbohydrates, which forces your body into ketosis and, thus, a reduction of body fats. This diet helps you lose fat and ensures the mass of the muscles is well preserved. Ketogenic diets promote weight loss through an increase in intake of protein, which has numerous weight-loss advantages. The diet regulates carbohydrates' consumption, which is a crucial component in weight loss and burning calories as a result of the conversion of proteins and fats into ketone bodies that run your organization. The diet also assists in burning fats rapidly while taking part in physical exercises, during rests, and other ordinary days to day activities.

Control of Glucose in the Body

Another advantage of adopting the diet is that it can lower and regulate your blood sugar levels. Carbohydrates are responsible for the rise of blood sugar levels in your blood, and thus that threat is eliminated once you start on the Ketogenic diet. The Ketogenic Pescatarian Diet is known for its ability to reduceHbA1c – a known measure of your blood glucose control. This measure is significantly reduced by the diet of people who have type 2 diabetes.

The diet is also useful to the other types of diabetes, such as type 1 diabetes or LADA, and thus the diet should also regulate the glucose in your blood. It is important to note that if the food is maintained, the chances of controlling your blood's glucose could help reduce the risk of any other health complications from occurring.

A Reduction in Reliance on the Medication-Related to Diabetes

As you have already been aware of the diet's ability to reduce blood sugar levels, the menu also offers a chance to patients who have type 2 diabetes to reduce their reliance on medication. After a good while of sticking to it, the list will pay your efforts as you will be able to do away with the drug-related to type 2 diabetes, a study found. You could ultimately come off your medicine, or the diet could help reduce your dosage. However, consult with your doctor first before doing away with the mediation.

Control of High Blood Pressure

Numerous people in the world today are living and surviving with high blood pressure. With high blood pressure, your body becomes prone to several ailments, such as heart-related diseases, kidney-related diseases, or even stroke. The Ketogenic Pescatarian Diet helps you reduce the risk of all these diseases because the diet decreases your body's blood pressure levels if you are overweight or suffering from type 2 diabetes.

An improved Mental Performance

The diet will significantly improve your ability to remember and recall and improve your ability to focus. Ingestion of foods such as salmon, which are Keto-friendly, could boost your mood and your learning abilities in the classroom setting. The diet could also help enhance your long-term memory.

Restoration of Insulin Sensitivity

The Ketogenic Pescatarian Diet is known for removing the cause of insulin resistance as a consequence of elevated insulin levels in your body. The diet cuts on the ingestion of carbohydrates, leading to high levels of insulin in the body. With a reduction of insulin level in your body, the chances of burning fat in your body increases. This is because elevated levels of insulin interfere with the breaking down of fats.

Improved Cholesterol Levels

The Ketogenic Pescatarian Diet is a great agent in ensuring that your cholesterol levels in your blood are regulated. However, it is recommended to let your doctor of physician put you on the Keto diet if you intend to regulate your body's cholesterol levels. This is because this topic on cholesterol is complicated and would require qualified personnel to handle.

Satiety

The diet is also known for its ability to have a positive effect on your appetite. The moment your body succeeds in getting into ketosis, it becomes more comfortable with burning fats, which could, in turn, force your body to stop craving for food and thus improving your chances of doing away with overeating. In the long end, you would most likely succeed in losing weight.

Benefits to Individuals with Diabetes

Diabetes is a result of raised blood sugar levels, which, over time, are harmful to the heart, kidneys, nerves, and blood vessels. Diabetes manifests when the body is not in a position to produce adequate insulin, and if your body becomes tough to insulin. The diet comes in and eliminates this possibility. Ketogenic diets are essential in curbing type 2 diabetes, the most experienced type of diabetes among adults because the diet helps you shed extra fat, which is associated with this site type of diabetes. As a result of adapting to the menu for long periods, you could get off your medication.

26. Disadvantages of Keto Diet

Along with the dramatic change in diet, there may be some negative experiences on the ketogenic diet. One of the more common issues is keto flu. This is a general feeling of fatigue that may accompany entering ketosis. This feeling of tiredness may be accompanied by nausea and upset stomach. It is a common reaction to the body as it adapts to reduced carbohydrates and the switch to getting energy from ketones instead of glucose.

Besides the keto flu, there may also be keto diarrhea. This is likely caused by the gallbladder producing more bile to deal with increased fat consumption. Until the body adjusts to the increased amounts of fat and enters ketosis, diarrhea may be a side effect. Diarrhea may also result from a reduction in the number of fiber ingested because of a decrease in carbohydrate consumption. The tissue from carbs must be replaced with tissue from low-carb vegetables. This will help mitigate diarrhea issues resulting from the lack of carbohydrates and, therefore, the fiber in the diet.

One way to reduce gastrointestinal issues associated with the keto diet is to make sure you drink plenty of water. It is essential to stay hydrated and flush out your system. Drinking lots of water helps to remove toxins from the body before they have time to linger in organs and tissues.

The keto diet will precipitate weight loss. Unfortunately, this weight loss may include the reduction of muscle mass as well as fat. This is not ideal, especially for women over 50 in whom muscle mass begins to atrophy naturally. Additionally, reduced muscle mass may change your metabolism because you burn more calories with muscle than fat. This loss of tissue is more likely to happen if you are consuming more fat than protein. The type of fat consumed will be essential to retain muscle mass as you lose weight.

13.   THE BEST WAYS TO LOSE WEIGHT FAST

There are many ways you can approach losing weight. What is required is consistency and commitment. If you have been on a diet before, you will know that it will take a while to see results. This time to see your results will only lengthen as you age. Losing weight is not a race. It is a marathon.

27. Eat Out Less

Kirsten David, a dietitian with Edu Plated, explained that we are more prone to weight gain as we grow old. As mentioned in the, our metabolism slows down, and we undergo hormone change.

This sounds like a no-brainer, but you may be eating out more than you think. Other than the fact that you may be unwittingly digesting the food that dials your blood sugar to eleven, eating out is common among older adults, starting from age 50.

Due to mental, physical, or social barriers, you may be prevented from losing weight effectively. Many people at this age are either too mentally or physically tired to cook at home themselves. Plus, there are no more children in the house as they would be living on their elsewhere.

Without having any mouths to feed other than your own, going out and eating seems quite practical, right? Don't have to worry about thinking of what you should prepare for dinner, or having to stress about doing the dishes. But in reality, letting others control what you put into your mouth is one of the first mistakes in dieting. You put yourself at risk of consuming a higher amount of processed foods and high-fat foods.

Even for people in their 20's, eating the wrong food will get them fat quickly. At your age, the consequence of weight gain will increase drastically.

Instead, plan your meal. We will discuss how you can do that and which dishes to incorporate into your diet to help you lose weight, what to avoid.

28. Don't Skip Meals

On the flip side, skipping meals also leads to weight gain. Diet oversimplified would be "Eat less, move more," but you will not get the full effect. The statement is not accurate because you need to know exactly what food you need to cut down and what activity to partake.

In this case, let us talk about skipping meals. This leads to a drop in metabolism because when your body senses that you are not getting any food, it goes into power-saving mode.

As we age, our hormones change as well. Estrogen and testosterone, in particular, are affected, and this causes your body to process sugar efficiently. However, if you skip meals, your body will lack the critical nutrients needed, such as calories and protein.

Providing your body with enough calories or protein will maintain your muscle mass and regulate your hormones. Without them, your internal system will go haywire, and it won't be easy to steer everything back on track.

If it is inconvenient, then you do not have to eat three meals a day. So long as you get enough calories and nutrients every day, you should be fine. Avoid snacking because you won't be losing any weight when you graze on food all day long. Other than that, make sure to stay hydrated with fluids such as tea, water, or coffee.

29. Eat Less at Night

Some people have the habit of having dinner right before bedtime. Not only does that interfere with your body's digestion process, but you will also get the lower quality sleep that you need at your age. Many studies have shown that consuming fewer calories at night could help you maintain a slimmer, fitter body and shed excess fat.

You also put yourself at risk of developing metabolic syndrome, which can lead to heart disease, diabetes, and stroke because of your high blood sugar level and excess body fat.

So, keep most of the calories for breakfast and lunch. Keep dinner light to help you sleep tight.

30. Sleep

As mentioned before, sleep plays a huge role in hormone regulation, among other weight-related bodily functions. The key to getting enough sleep is establishing an asleep and morning routine. Do not look at blue lights (fluorescent, phone, computer) for at least 30 minutes before you go to sleep. If you must, you can download some applications for your device to make it produce orange light instead of blue. Orange lights are easier on your eyes and do not disrupt sleep.

31. Team Up

Getting into a new eating pattern or daily routine can be a challenge. Staying motivated requires even more willpower. Therefore, getting your friend, co-worker, or a family member to take up this new routine might give you a better chance to stick to your plan and achieve your goals. Try Intermittent Fasting

Intermittent fasting is well-known because it does not change what you eat, but when and how often you do. Ditch the juice cleanses. The most common form is called the 16/8, but you do not have to do that. Instead, try fasting-mimicking. This form of fasting has been proven to improve your health. People who have tried this diet plan reported that they have lost six pounds on average, shredded up to two inches off their waistline, and significantly lowered their cancer risk.

Fasting-mimicking works because the nerves in your hypothalamus are damaged as you gain weight. They are responsible for conducting signals from your fat cells to your brain. When they are damaged, your mind does not know when you have eaten your fill. Therefore, you are prone to overeating.

However, when you give yourself some time away from eating, you let your hypothalamic nerves to rest and recuperate. That is why fasting-mimicking requires you to allocate five days out of every month to eat just between 750 to 1,000 calories, well below the recommended daily calorie intake. It sounds terrible to starve yourself, but you need to give your nerves a break to reset themselves.

Start friendly and manageable by eating only 800 calories twice a week, and your calorie sources for those days are primarily from vegetables, protein, and healthy oils (olive oils).

Of course, your stomach will feel empty on those days. To help alleviate this problem, consider following a low-carb diet as you fast. Thirty percent of your calories should come from protein, non-starchy veggies, beans, and nuts.

The best time to eat starchy carbohydrates is at the very end of the meal after your fill of veggies and protein. Doing this helps lower your blood sugar level and insulin as well as an increase of hormones to help you feel full for longer.

Please, download Intermittent Fasting After 50, if you are interested.

32. Mindful Eating

Sometimes, you do not even need to make that many changes. All you need is to put your attention in the right place as you eat. Your weight gain may be caused by stress. If that is the case, then you may need to practice mindful eating.

You might be overeating just because you are stressed. Therefore, practicing mindfulness techniques can be very helpful to help alleviate your anxiety and make you aware of how much you are eating.

Those who have practiced this technique are more successful in their weight loss efforts. Mindful eating requires you to pay attention to how full or hungry you feel, meal planning, focusing solely on your food tastes, and not doing anything else when you eat (such as watching TV).

To get started, just eat slowly. Place your fork between bites and take your time chewing your food. Focus on how it tastes and do not watch TV, look at your phone, or do anything other than eating.

The trick behind mindful eating is that your body takes time to detect when it is full. If you eat quickly, you already overate by the time your body realizes it is complete. Plus, it would be best if you took the time to enjoy tasty meals that you cook for yourself and reinforce the belief that your healthy home-cooked food helps your body maintain its youth.

14. WEIGHT LOSS AFFIRMATIONS

An affirmation is any statement made to help you validate the thoughts that you need to retrain how you think. Throughout our lives, we may start to use unhealthy affirmations, such as "I'll start on Monday" or "I'll do it later." These thoughts become natural to us, eventually creating the way that we live.

Include the healthy affirmations below in your life as often as possible to turn around the patterns of thinking that have made you want to change yourself.

We've split such affirmations into three, inclusive of the most important words of wisdom that you need in your daily life. These are all phrases that you should say to yourself as often as possible. As we read them, let them flow through your mind as if they are your own.

Write the words down to remember them further, put notes around your house with the affirmations written on them, or simply find other creative ways to incorporate them into your life. Let's start reading them now so that you can get these ideas in your head right away.

Dedication Affirmations

I am dedicated mostly to myself.

I put my health first before anything else in my life.

I am dedicated to healthy living, not any other form of life.

I am mindful of the things that I put into my body.

I make sure that I am consistently working out for my health.

I am always looking for ways to grow.

When I say that I am going to do something, I do my best to stick to it.

It feels good to be dedicated.

I am a passionate person.

Once I set my mind to something, I know what I need to do to achieve that.

I am happy when I am dedicated.

I am healthy when I am happy.

I am only focused on adding as much health as possible in my life.

I am focused on reality and how I can be happy all the time.

Everything becomes more manageable when I am dedicated.

It feels better to say 'yes' to my present self than to say 'no' to my future self.

I am always looking out for what will be the best in the future.

I am always looking for new ways to improve my health.

I am highly aware of how I can consistently boost my health.

I only add things that are good for me.

I treat myself when I need to, but I am always dedicated to being healthy so that I can quickly get back on track.

I find motivation even when I don't want to do much of anything at all.

I find ways to include better health in every aspect of my life.

I heal myself with the choices that I make.

I will always remain loyal to my health.

Self–Control Affirmations

I am patient and willing to wait for results.

I know what I need, as well as what I have to say 'no' to.

I understand what is right and wrong for me.

I am focused on practicing discipline.

I appreciate what I already have.

I do not act on impulse.

I think before I push through with a decision.

I am more durable than the biggest craving that I may feel throughout the day.

I am proud of my ability to display self-control.

I take everything in one at a time, accepting and appreciating everything that is around me.

Even the struggle is something that I am appreciative of.

I can conquer my own most prominent feelings of wanting to eat more and more.

I do not allow myself to binge eat or partake in other unhealthy patterns of eating.

I do not give into temporary urges.

I trust myself and my ability to be disciplined.

I know what I need more of and what I can do just fine with what is already there.

My temptation does not easily influence me.

I do not wait for good things to come; I take actionable steps to get them myself.

I understand that the best time to finish something is right after starting it.

I believe in my ability to make the best decisions for my health.

I don't put things off.

I do not allow procrastination in my life.

I have control over my most significant wants and desires.

I am focused only on achieving my goals.

I look out for my future self and make the best decisions with them in mind.

Healthy Living Affirmations

I can make myself feel better.

There are no outside sources that I need just to improve my health.

I do not allow anything else to make me feel unhealthy.

I know that healthy living starts in my mind.

I understand how healthy living will improve my soul.

I can feel good whenever I want.

I choose to do things that are best for my health.

I deserve to have a healthy life.

Healthy habits come naturally to me, the more I decide to let them into my body.

I am in control of the habits that I have in my life.

I am aware of the small decisions I make that can affect my health.

I understand the minor things that I can improve for the big picture of my health.

I am aware of how I need to improve my health to be able to live better.

I have a positive attitude when it comes to improving my health.

I can sacrifice certain things if it means I can start living healthier.

I am confident in my ability to know what is best for my health overall.

Each decision I make to become healthier makes me feel better.

Others see my healthy habits, and it can help encourage theirs, too.

I am excited to seek healthy habits because I know that it will help make my life better.

I always have my health at the center of my focus at the end of the day.

I am not scared of what may happen as I change my habits.

I am in control of whether I am going to live a healthy life or not.

I am dedicated to making the best decisions possible for my health.

15.   10 TASTY AND HEALTHY RECIPES

1. Salmon Skewers

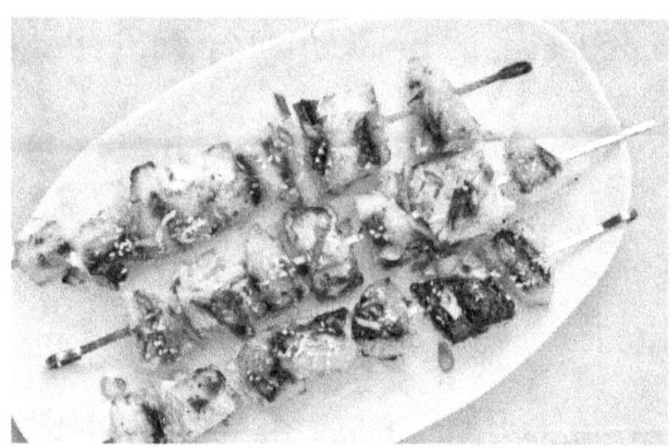

Preparation Time: 35 mins
Cooking Time: 30 mins
Servings: 4
Ingredients:

- ¼ c fresh spinach, chopped fine
- 1 lb. salmon cut into bite-sized pieces
- ¼ t black pepper freshly ground - ½ t pink Himalayan salt - 1 T olive oil
- 3½ oz sliced prosciutto
- 1 c full-fat mayonnaise
- Eight wooden or metal skewers

Directions:

1. Heat oven to 400 degrees.
2. Mix olive oil spinach salt and pepper in a 1-gallon storage bag.
3. Coat salmon pieces in oil mixture by placing them in the bag.

4. Place salmon on skewers.
5. Wrap salmon skewers with prosciutto.
6. Bake salmon for approximately 15 minutes, turning every 3 or 4 minutes.
7. When prosciutto is crispy, and salmon is cooked, remove from oven.
8. Serve with mayonnaise on the side.

33. **Nutrition:**
34. **Calories:** 680
35. **Carbohydrates:** 1g
36. **Protein:** 28g
37. **Fat:** 62g
38. **Sodium:** 1092 mg

2. Coconut Salmon with Napa Cabbage

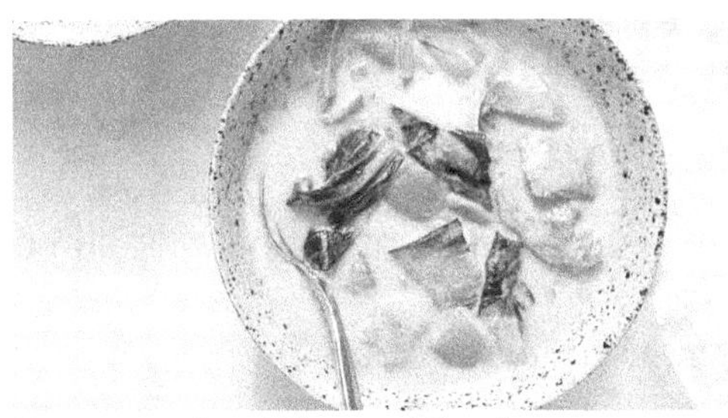

Preparation Time: 45 mins
Cooking Time: 40 mins
Servings: 4
Ingredients:

- 1¼ lbs. salmon - 1 T olive oil
- ½ c unsweetened shredded coconut
- 1 t turmeric
- 1 t kosher salt

- ½ t garlic powder
- 4 T olive oil, for frying
- 2 c. Napa cabbage
- One stick butter
- Salt and pepper

Directions:

1. Cut salmon into small 1-inch chunks.
2. Grind coconut to make it more likely to stay on the fish pieces. If you don't have a grinder, use a sharp knife to chop the shredded coconut as finely as possible.
3. Mix coconut, turmeric, salt, and garlic powder in a bowl. In another dish, coat salmon with one tablespoon of olive oil.
4. Take Dredge oil-coated salmon in dry ingredients. Heat 4 tablespoons of olive oil in a frying pan to medium heat.
5. Cook coconut coated salmon until crispy. It will take about one minute per side. Make sure each team gets nicely browned.
6. Remove cooked salmon from the pan and keep warm while cooking the cabbage.
7. Slice cabbage into thin strips with a knife or shred in a food processor.
8. Melt butter in pan used to cook salmon.
9. Cook cabbage until tender.
10. Season cabbage with salt and pepper.
11. Serve cabbage with salmon and enjoy it.

Nutrition:

Calories: 744

Carbohydrates: 3g

Protein: 32g

Fat: 67g

Sodium: 1457 mg

3. Keto Tuna Casserole

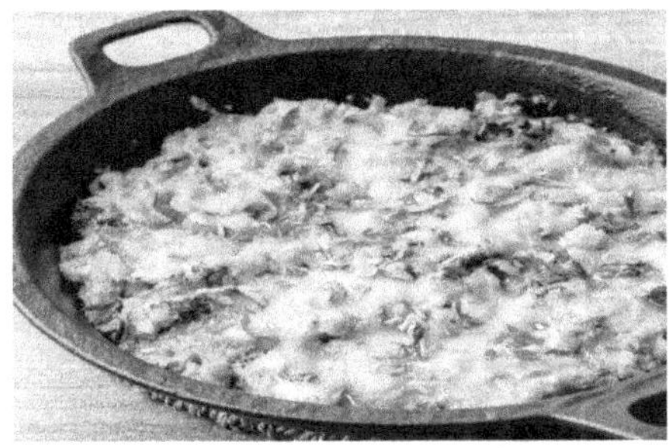

Preparation Time: 45 mins
Cooking Time: 40 mins
Servings: 4
Ingredients:
- 4 T butter
- 2 T olive oil
- One medium onion, diced
- One green bell pepper, diced
- Five celery stalks, diced
- 2 c baby spinach chopped fine
- Two large cans tuna in olive oil, drained
- 1 c mayonnaise
- 1 ½ c freshly shredded Parmesan cheese
- 1 t red pepper flakes
- Salt and pepper

Directions:
1. Preheat oven to 350 degrees.
2. Heat butter and olive oil in a large skillet.
3. Sauté onions, green bell pepper, celery, and spinach in butter/oil.

4. In a bowl, mix tuna, Parmesan cheese, mayonnaise, and red pepper flake until thoroughly combined.
5. Add sautéed vegetables to the tuna mixture and stir until everything is incorporated
6. Pour tuna mixture into a casserole dish for baking.
7. Bake in the oven for 30 minutes.
8. Remove casserole from the oven when golden brown on top and bubbly.

Nutrition:
Calories: 953
Carbohydrates: 5g
Protein: 43g
Fat: 83g
Sodium: 1376 mg

4. Baked Fish Fillets with Vegetables in Foil

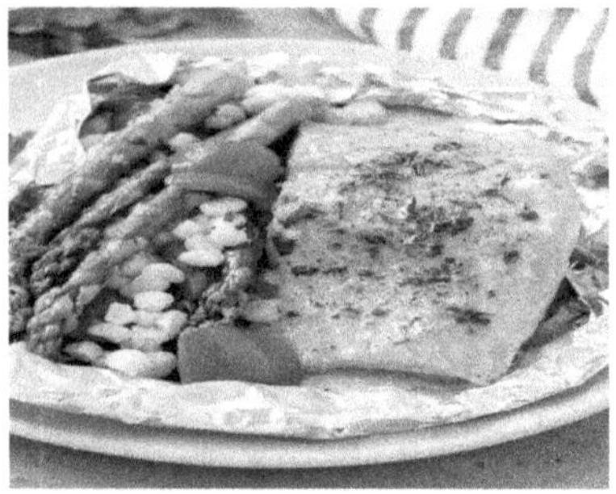

Preparation time: 10 minutes
Cooking time: 40 minutes
Servings: 3
Ingredients:
- 1 lb. cod (or any white fish)
- One red bell pepper, sliced
- Six cherry tomatoes halved

- One leek (small size, only the white part, sliced)
- ¼ onion, sliced
- ½ zucchini, sliced
- One clove garlic, chopped
- 2 tbsp olives
- 1 oz butter
- 2 tbsp olive oil
- ½ lemon sliced to taste
- Coriander leaves, to taste (optional)
- Salt and pepper to taste

Directions:

1. Preheat oven to 400°F.
2. Slice the zucchini, leek, onion, bell pepper and lemon, cut tomatoes in half, chop the garlic.
3. Transfer all the vegetables to a baking sheet lined with foil.
4. Cut the fish into bite-sized pieces and add to the vegetables. Add salt and pepper, drizzle olive oil and add slices of butter around evenly.
5. Fold the foil and make sure you seal the joints of the foil tightly.
6. Bake for 35 – 40 minutes.
7. It can be served with aioli or any other low carb sauce of your choice.

Nutrition:
Calories: 339
Fat: 19g
Protein: 35g
Carbs: 5g
Sodium: 569 mg

5. Baked Salmon with Almonds and Cream Sauce

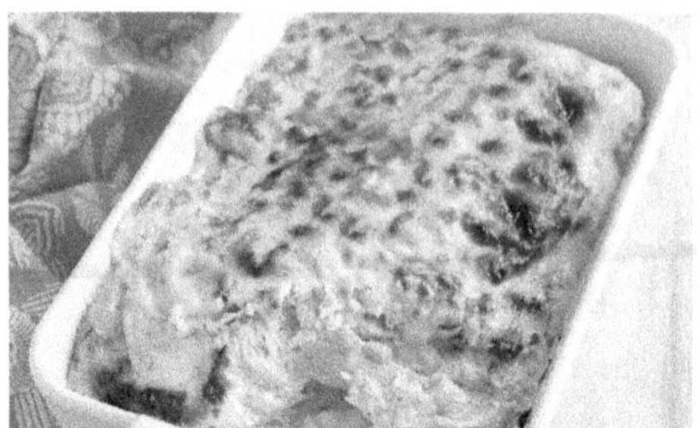

Preparation time: 10 minutes
Cooking time: 20 minutes
Servings: 2
Ingredients:

- Almond Crumbs Creamy Sauce
- 3 tbsp shaved almonds
- 2 tbsp almond milk (for thinning the sauce if necessary)
- ½ cup cream cheese
- Salt to taste
- Fish
- One salmon fillet (about ½ lb.)
- 1 tsp coconut oil
- 1 tbsp lemon zest
- 1 tsp salt
- White pepper to taste

Directions:

1. Prepare the salmon: cut the salmon in half. Mix the lemon zest, salt, and pepper and rub the mixture on the salmon. Let it cook in the refrigerator for 20 minutes so the seasonings will be absorbed. Meanwhile, preheat the oven to 300°F.

2. Heat some coconut oil on a nonstick baking dish. Fry the fish on both sides for a few minutes and make sure that the fish is sealed. Top with almond crumbs and bake in the oven for 10 to 15 minutes.
3. Take the dish out of the oven and transfer the fish to a separate plate. Set aside.
4. Place the baking dish on fire and add the cream cheese. Combine the fish cooking juices and the cheese for a more flavorful sauce.
5. Mix well until uniformed. If necessary, add some almond milk to the sauce.
6. Pour the sauce onto the fish. Best served hot.

Nutrition:
Calories 522
Fat 44g
Protein 28g
Carbs 2.4g
Sodium 1432 mg

6. Spring Greens Soup

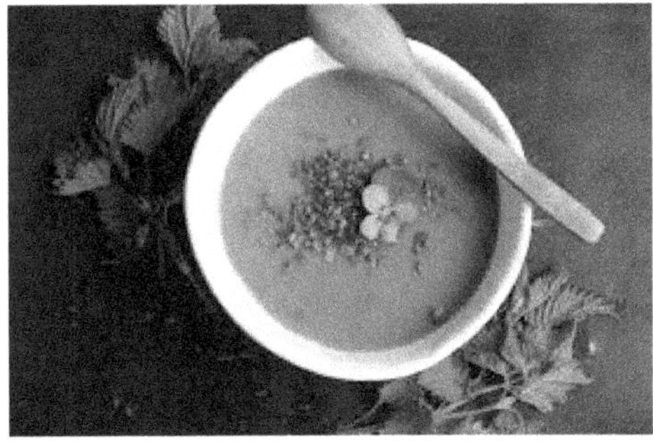

Preparation time: 10 minutes

Cooking time: 30 minutes

Servings: 4

Ingredients:

- Mustard greens – Two cups, chopped
- Collard greens – Two cups, chopped
- Vegetable stock – Four cups
- Onion – 1, chopped
- Salt and ground black pepper to taste
- Coconut amino – Two Tbsp.
- Fresh ginger – 2 tsp. grated

1.

Directions:

1. Put the stock altogether into a saucepan and bring to a simmer over medium heat.
2. Add ginger, coconut aminos, salt, pepper, onion, mustard, and collard greens. Stir, cover, and cook for 30 minutes. Remove from the heat.
3. Blend the soup with a hand mixer.
4. Serve.

Nutrition:

Calories: 35

Fat: 1g

Carb: 7g

Protein: 2g

Sodium: 64 mg

7. Celery Soup

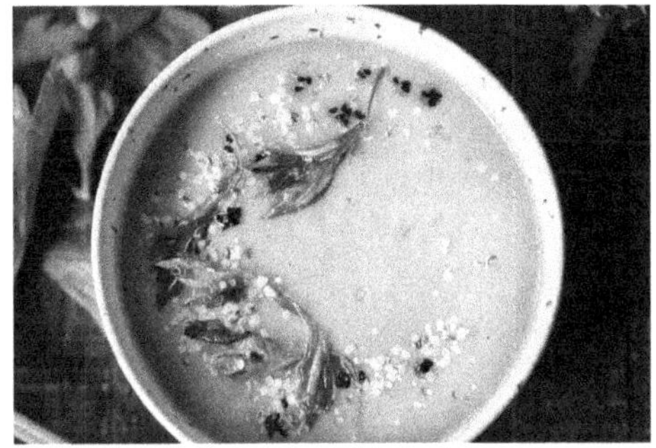

Preparation time: 10 minutes
Cooking time: 30 minutes
Servings: 6
Ingredients:
- Celery – 1 bunch, chopped
- Onion – 1, chopped
- Green onion – 1 bunch, chopped
- Garlic cloves – 4, minced
- Salt and ground black pepper to taste
- Parsley – 1 fresh bunch, chopped
- Fresh mint bunches – 2, chopped
- Persian lemons – 3 dried, pricked with a fork
- Water – 2 cups
- Olive oil – 4 Tbsp.

Directions:
1. Heat a saucepan with oil over medium heat.
2. Add onion, garlic, and green onions. Stir and cook for 6 minutes.
3. Add Persian lemons, celery, salt, pepper, water, stir, cover pan, and simmer on medium heat for 20 minutes.
4. Add parsley and mint, stir, and cook for 10 minutes.
5. Blend with a hand mixer and serve.

Nutrition:
Calories: 100
Fat: 9.5g
Carb: 4.4g
Protein: 1g
Sodium: 55 mg

8. Eggplant Stew

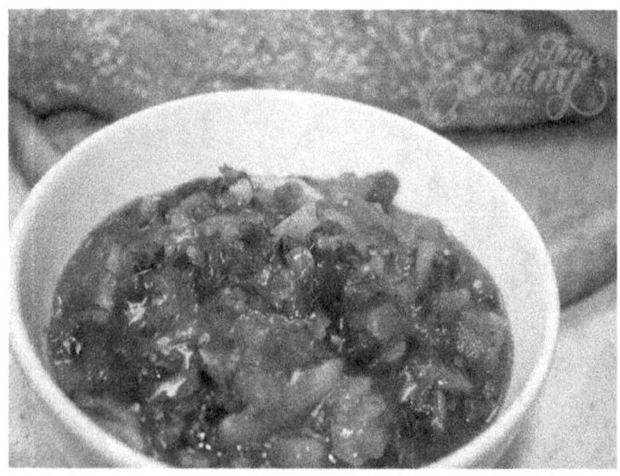

Preparation time: 10 minutes
Cooking time: 30 minutes
Servings: 4
Ingredients:

- Onion – 1, chopped - Garlic – 2 cloves, chopped - Fresh parsley – 1 bunch, chopped
- Salt and black pepper to taste
- Dried oregano – 1 tsp.
- Eggplants – 2, cut into chunks
- Olive oil – 2 Tbsp.
- Capers – 2 Tbsp. chopped
- Green olives – 12, pitted and sliced

- Tomatoes – 5, chopped
- Herb vinegar – 3 Tbsp.

Directions:

1. In a saucepan
2. heat oil over medium heat.
3. Add oregano, eggplant, salt, pepper, and stir-fry for 5 minutes.
4. Add parsley, onion, garlic, and stir-fry for 4 minutes.
5. Add tomatoes, vinegar, olives, capers, and stir-fry for 15 minutes.
6. Adjust seasoning and stir.
7. Serve.

Nutrition:
Calories: 280
Fat: 17.9g
Carb: 8.4g
Protein: 5.4g
Sodium: 308 mg

9. Asparagus Frittata

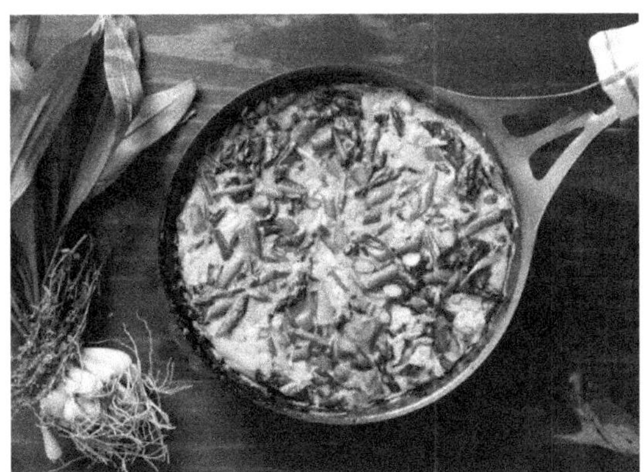

Preparation time: 10 minutes
Cooking time: 15 minutes
Servings: 4
Ingredients:

- Onion – ¼ cup, chopped
- A drizzle of olive oil
- Asparagus spears – One-pound, cut into one-inch pieces
- Salt and ground black pepper to taste
- Eggs – four, whisked
- Cheddar cheese – One cup, grated

Directions:

1. Heat a pan with oil over medium heat.
2. Add onions and stir-fry for 3 minutes.
3. Add asparagus and stir-fry for 6 minutes.
4. Add eggs and stir-fry for 3 minutes.
5. Add salt, pepper, and sprinkle with cheese.
6. Broil for 3 minutes and place it on the oven.
7. Divide frittata between plates and serve.

Nutrition:
Calories: 202
Fat: 13.3g
Carb: 5.8g
Protein: 15.1g
Sodium: 106 mg

10. Bell Peppers Soup

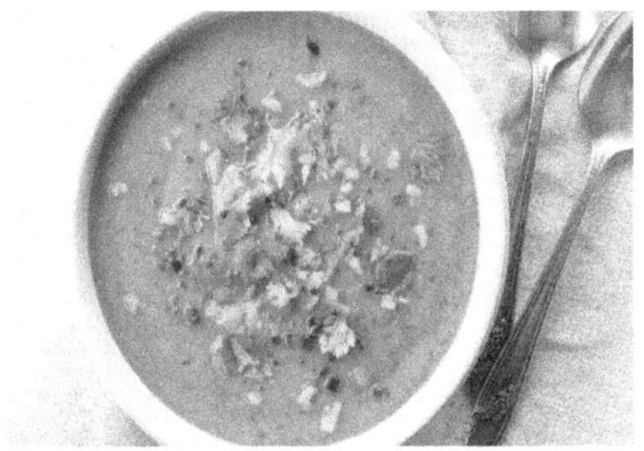

Preparation time: 10 minutes
Cooking time: 15 minutes
Servings: 6
Ingredients:

- Roasted bell peppers – 12, seeded and chopped
- Olive oil – 2 tbsp. - Garlic – 2 cloves, minced - Vegetable stock – 30 ounces
- Salt and black pepper to taste - Water - 6 ounces
- Heavy cream – 2/3 cup
- Onion – 1, chopped
- Parmesan cheese – ¼ cup, grated
- Celery stalks – 2, chopped

Directions:

1. Heat a saucepan with oil over medium heat.
2. Add onion, garlic, celery, salt, and pepper. Stir-fry for 8 minutes.
3. Add water, bell peppers, stock, stir, and bring to a boil.
4. Simmer for 5 minutes and cover it up and let it be.
5. Remove from heat and blend with a hand mixer.
6. Then adjust seasoning, and add cream. Stir and bring to a boil.
7. Remove from the heat and serve on bowls.

8. Sprinkle with Parmesan and serve.

Nutrition:
Calories: 155
Fat: 12g
Carb: 8.6g
Protein: 4.7g
Sodium: 90 mg

16. TOP TIPS AND CAUTIONS FOR GOING AND STAYING PESCATARIAN ON THE KETOGENIC PESCATARIAN DIET

There are so many incredibly delicious foods out there that are healthy, plant-based, and keto-friendly. When Pescatarian starts to implement this diet, there are a few tricks to help you on your keto journey with minimal effort. Here are some of the best tips you should follow:

39. Get Your Carbs From Vegetables

While carbs are limited on the keto diet, you will need to consume a healthy amount of low-carb vegetables to supply yourself with sufficient bulk and fiber to keep your stomach full. I encourage all Pescatarian s to explore and open themselves up to new sorts of vegetables cooked in different ways. If eating vegetables raw doesn't seem tasty, try cooking the vegetables with butter or coconut oil with plenty of seasoning. Here are some low-carb vegetables you will be eating:

- Kale
- Collard Greens
- Spinach
- Swiss Chard
- Asparagus
- Lettuce
- Green Beans
- Broccoli
- Cucumber
- Summer Squash
- Winter Squash
- White Cabbage
- Red Cabbage

- Cauliflower
- Bell Peppers
- Onions
- Mushrooms
- Tomatoes
- Garlic
- Eggplants

40. Get Plenty Of Sleep

Establishing healthy sleep habits on a Ketogenic Pescatarian Diet will help you go to sleep faster and wake up feeling rejuvenated. Research also shows that not getting enough sleep can significantly hinder your ability to lose weight and increase your levels of stress hormones. With that said, you must prioritize sleep! If you are finding it hard to go to sleep, try taking natural sleep aids such as melatonin, which can work miracles.

41. Lower Your Stress

If you are suffering from chronic stress, it will interfere with your body's ability to achieve ketosis. This is because stress hormones raise your blood sugar levels, which thwarts your body's strength from burning fat for fuel. After all, there is too much glucose in your bloodstream. If you are currently going through a phase of high stress in your life, it's recommended you avoid the keto diet until you can keep the pressure at bay. You should start the keto diet when you can effectively fight off stress and commit a large portion of your time towards maintaining the state of ketosis. If you are currently dealing with stress in your life, it's still possible for you to follow the keto Pescatarian diet. All you need to do is take proper steps to reduce the amounts of stress in your life, which includes getting sufficient sleep hours, regular exercise, or practicing relaxation techniques such as deep breathing, meditation, or yoga.

42. Increase Your Salt Intake

A widely believed misconception is that our sodium intake should be deficient, but this is generally only an issue on high carb diets. This is because high carbohydrate diets raise your insulin levels. When insulin levels are too high, your kidney begins to retain sodium rather than extreme them. Adopting the keto diet means your insulin levels will be low, and your body excretes more salt since no carbs are dwelling in your body to spike insulin and retain sodium. Once you are in ketosis, it is recommended you add three to five grams of sodium in your diet. This will help avoid electrolyte imbalance. The best ways to ensure you get enough salt in your diet are:

Drinking homemade organic bone broth each day.

Sprinkling a little more salt onto your meals.

Adding salt to your drinking water throughout your day.

Eating salted nuts

Eating foods that naturally contain sodium, such as celery or cucumbers.

43. Engage In Physical Activity

Frequent exercises while on the Ketogenic Pescatarian Diet can increase your ketone levels and help you transition into ketosis much more smoothly. To achieve ketosis, your body needs to get rid of any remaining glucose in your body. Exercising uses various types of energy for fuel, including carbs, fats, and amino acids. The more you apply, the faster your body uses up its glycogen stores. Once your body completely depletes its glycogen storages, it will find alternative forms of fuel and will turn to fat for energy through the metabolic state of ketosis. Ensure to include a workout regimen that incorporates both high-intensity exercises in concurrent with low-intensity steady-state activities like walking or jogging. This will help you elevate your blood sugar levels and help your body in entering ketosis.

44. Keep Track Of Your Carb Macronutrients

Counting your carbohydrate intake is critical for the success of the ketogenic diet. Be sure to do your best in avoiding hidden carbs and hidden sugars in foods that appear to be keto-friendly but are not. Some examples are
Chicken wings loaded with buffalo sauce or barbecue sauce
Milk
Most fruits (berries are fine only in small quantities)
Breaded meats
Pre-packaged meals and processed foods
If you are following the Ketogenic Pescatarian Diet and the Pescatarian diet, you need to make it a habit to carefully observe the nutrition label of everything you eat until you understand the foods to avoid. The maximum amount of carbohydrates on the keto Pescatarian diet is 50 grams. When figuring out your carb count, you want to look for your daily net carb intake. To calculate your net carbs, follow the equation:
Total carbs - Fiber = Net Carbs
The rule of thumb is to have a 20 to 30 intake of net carbs per day. If you frequently exercise, you can get away with more and still maintain ketosis.

45. Clean Your Kitchen

You can increase your success on this diet if you only have access to healthy plant-based, keto-friendly foods in your kitchen. Many people fail on this diet due to having carb-packed meals lying around in their pantry. Cleaning out your kitchen and pantry of all unfriendly keto foods such as sugar, all-purpose flour, bread, pasta, soda, candy, rice, and legumes will force you to stick to the Pescatarian keto diet to the end. This may sound a little bit extreme, but to stay on track, you need to replace all your carb foods with keto-friendly foods.

46. Have Quick Meals Ready

The key to success with any diet is sticking with it. Unfortunately, mistakes are bound to happen in even our best-laid plans. There may be days where you simply can't follow the keto diet. For instance, if you are traveling and don't have time to cook, or if you are going out to eat with friends or family. For those certain occasions when you can't cook keto meals, and you need something quick to get you going, here are some easy ideas:

Keto Butter Coffee (mix one tablespoon of MCT oil and one tablespoon of butter with 1 cup of black brewed coffee)

Eat a couple of tablespoons of nut butter

Add some coconut oil or MCT oil to your morning cup of coffee or tea

Eat some dark chocolate or cheese throughout the day.

47. Be Mindful When Eating Out

Eating out while on the Pescatarian keto diet can be tricky. When eating out for dinner, here are a couple of ideas:

Find the restaurant website online and look at the menu ahead of time to know what is keto-compliant.

Avoid carb-packed foods such as pasta and rice dishes.

Avoid breaded and fried foods

Avoid desserts

When ordering salads, choose olive oil or vinegar rather than sugary dressings or ranch.

Tell the waiter that you are on the keto Pescatarian diet and if there are any plant-based, keto-friendly meals you can order.

The longer you follow the keto Pescatarian diet, the better you will get at recognizing keto-friendly foods. It will take some time and practice, but you will get the gist of it.

48. Try Meal Prepping

One of the hardest things about the keto diet is sticking to it, and meal prep makes the road easier. Think about the many times you tried diets but never have easily accessible meals ready. Meal prep can turn your refrigerator to a grab-and-go dispensator in which you can save yourself time and money, especially if you are a busy person. For some people, meal prepping can simply mean chopping your ingredients ahead of time that will be cooked later. It can also mean rationing out elements before the actual cooking process. Commonly, people prepare all the meals they plan to eat for the weak in a single day and store them inside their refrigerator.

When meal prepping, the key is always to plan. Make a list of all the meals you want to eat for the week and purchase the ingredients at the grocery accordingly beforehand. Then, you can dedicate yourself a single day to cook your meals and properly store them.

17.   CONCLUSION

How long can I be on the Pescatarian ketogenic diet? Is it safe for the long-term? Many people and cultures go into ketosis and stay there for a long time without any adverse effects. Depending on your health goals, your practitioner may recommend a specific

 period for you to be on the ketogenic diet. Many people and cultures go into ketosis and stay there for a long time without any adverse effects.

Pescatarian ketogenic diet slims down have sincerely gone beforehand substantial in the preceding 18 months, and all matters considered. It's an unusual approach to shed those undesirable pounds brisk, but additionally, a brilliant method to get healthful and remain as such. For people who have attempted the Keto Diet are nevertheless on it; it's something aside from a consuming regimen. It's a lifestyle, a very new lifestyle. Be that as it may, much like any sizable shift in our lives, it is anything, however, a simple one, it takes a mind-boggling degree of obligation and assurance.

Bravo, But now not for all? - Although a ketogenic weight-reduction plan has been utilized to exceptionally improve individuals'satisfaction, there are some out there who do not share the more significant component's perspective. In any case, for what cause is that precisely? As a long way as we can don't forget, we were endorsed that the excellent manner of disposing of the extra weight was to stop eating the fat-filled nourishments that we're so acquainted with eating each day. So schooling individuals to consume healthful fat (The catchphrase is Healthy), you could realize why a few people would be suspicious approximately how and why you would devour progressively fat to accomplish weight loss and achieve it quickly. This concept conflicts with all that we've got ever theory nearly weight loss.

Had been created by using the liver because of starvation or if the person pursued an ingesting regimen wealthy with excessive ats and extraordinarily low carbs. Later on that 12 months, a man from the Mayo Clinic through the name of Russel Wilder named it the "Ketogenic Diet," and applied it to treat epilepsy in small children with remarkable achievement. But because of headways in medication, it became supplanted.

My Struggles Starting Keto I started Keto February twenty-eighth, 2018, I had taken a stab at the Keto Diet once before round a half yr earlier, however, was usually unable to bear the first week. The first week on Keto is the most noticeably horrible piece of the entire procedure, that is when the feared Keto Flu indicates up likewise known as the carb flu. The average response you are frame studies when changing from consuming glucose (sugar) as vitality to ingesting fats. Numerous individuals who've gone on the Keto Diet say that it seems like pulling lower back from an addictive substance. This can remain anyplace between three days to a whole week; it just kept going more than one day for my situation.

Individuals who've had the keto Flu report feeling tired, throbbing, queasy, dazed, and have lousy headaches in addition to other matters. The most critical week is ordinary, while individuals endeavoring a Keto Diet falls flat and quit. Simply do not forget this takes place to absolutely everyone from the get-go all the at the same time as, and if you can move past the initial week, the hardest component is finished. There are more than one cures you can use to help you with overcoming this unpleasant spell. Taking Electrolyte supplements, closing hydrated, consuming bone juices, eating extra meat, and getting lots of rest. Keto Flu is a deplorable occasion that jumps out at each person as the body ousts the run of the mill's regular eating regimen.   You   simply need to govern through.

What Does A Ketogenic Pescatarian Diet Resemble? - When the healthy individual eats a feast wealthy in carbs, their body takes the ones carbs and changes over them into glucose for fuel. Glucose is the body's essential wellspring of gas while carbs are to be had within the body, on a Keto weight loss plan there are extremely low if any in any respect carbs gobbled which powers the authority to apply different   types   of   energy   to   hold the body working appropriately.   This   is   the place healthy fat becomes probably the   essential factor. With the nonattendance of carbs, the liver takes unsaturated lipids within

the organization and adjustments over them into ketone bodies.

Try no longer to devour higher than 20g of carbs every day to keep up the ordinary Ketogenic weight loss plan. I, for one, ate beneath 10g each day for an increasing number of extreme come across, but I accomplished my underlying objectives, to mention the very least. I lost 28 lbs. in a little beneath three weeks.

What Is Ketosis? When the body is energized absolutely by fat, it enters a nation called Ketosis," which is a function nation for the organization. After the whole thing of the sugars and unhealthy fat were expelled from the frame for the   duration   of   the   first   couple   of   weeks, the structure is currently unfastened, a   surprising spike in the call for wholesome fat. Ketosis has several potential benefits identified with rapid weight loss, health, or execution. In specific circumstances like sort one diabetes, inordinate ketosis can become very risky, wherein as in precise instances, mixed with discontinuous fasting may be amazingly useful for people experiencing kind two diabetes. Significant paintings are being led on this factor via Dr. Jason Fung, M.D. (Nephrologist) of the Intensive Dietary Management Program.

What I Can and Can't Eat - For another man or woman to Keto, it very well may be seeking to adhere to a low-carb diet, despite the reality that fat is the foundation of this consuming routine try not to consume all kinds of fats. Healthy fat is essential, but what are healthful fats you could inquire. Healthy fat would include grass-strengthened meats (sheep, hamburger, goat, venison), wild got fish and fish, fed red meat, and poultry. Eggs and salt-free portions of margarine can likewise be ingested. Make positive to keep away from bland vegetables, herbal products, and grains. Prepared nourishments are not the slightest bit recounted in any form or structure on the Ketogenic food plan; synthetic sugars and milk can likewise represent a severe issue.

I would like to thank you for purchasing this book and taking the time to read it. I hope that it has been helpful to you!

The Ketogenic Pescatarian diet is very beneficial for your health and stamina. Combining these two diets is one of the best you can find for your physical well-being and mental performance. Commit to it, and you will reap the benefits!

Did you like this book? Then don't forget to leave an on Amazon!

This way, other readers can get inspired too.

Do Not Go Yet, One Last Thing To Do
If you enjoyed this book or found it useful, I'd be very grateful if you'd post a short review on Amazon. Your support does make a difference, and I read all the reviews personally so I can get your feedback and make this book even better.
Thanks again for your support!